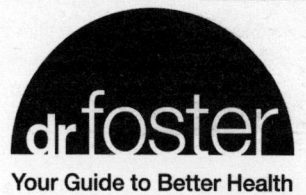

Your Guide to Better Health

DR FOSTER
GOOD CONSULTANT
GUIDE

1 3 5 7 9 10 8 6 4 2

Copyright © 2002 by Dr Foster Ltd

First published 2002 by Vermilion,
an imprint of Ebury Press, Random House,
20 Vauxhall Bridge Road, London SW1V 2SA
www.randomhouse.co.uk

Random House Australia (Pty) Limited
20 Alfred Street, Milsons Point, Sydney,
New South Wales 2061, Australia
Random House New Zealand Limited
18 Poland Road, Glenfield, Auckland 10, New Zealand
Random House South Africa (Pty) Limited
Endulini, 5a Jubilee Road, Parktown 2193, South Africa

The Random House Group Limited Reg. No. 954009

Papers used by Vermilion are natural, recyclable products made from wood grown in sustainable forests.

Printed and bound in Great Britain by
Bookmarque Ltd, Croydon, Surrey

A CIP catalogue record for this book is available
from the British Library

ISBN 0091883849

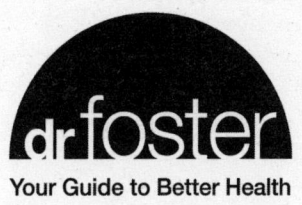

dr foster
Your Guide to Better Health

DR FOSTER
GOOD CONSULTANT
GUIDE

Researched by Dr Foster

Text by Rachel Gardner
Patsy Westcott and James Kinchen

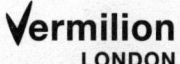

Vermilion
LONDON

Who is Dr Foster?

Dr Foster provides authoritative information on health services of all kinds in the UK. Our aim is to empower patients with information to help them access the best possible care. We are supervised by an independent Ethics committee that has legal powers to ensure that guides meet the highest standards and to investigate complaints.

The Ethics committee currently comprises the following membership:

Dr Jack Tinker, dean of the Royal Society of Medicine and chair of the committee

Sir Donald Irvine, past president, General Medical Council

Dr Michael Dixon, chair, NHS Alliance

Peter Griffiths, chief executive, Health Quality Service

Dianne Hayter, member of the board of the National Patient Safety Agency and the National Consumer Council

Professor Alan Maynard, director, Health Policy Unit, York University and chair, York Health Services NHS Trust

Wilma MacPherson, visiting professor at King's College London and a consultant in Health Services

Bridget Gill, head of communications, North and East Yorkshire & Northern Lincolnshire Strategic Health Authority

Trevor Campbell Davis, chief executive, Whittington Hospital

Douglas Webb, operations and development director, Friends of the Elderly

Vanessa Bourne, chair, Patients Association

Dr Philip Davies, medical director, Pontypridd and Rhondda NHS Trust

Professor Nairn Wilson, president of the General Dental Council.

Dr Foster Help at Hand

Dr Foster collects data on local hospital, maternity and fertility services. It also has comprehensive information on hospital doctors and complementary therapists. Call the **Help at Hand Service** on **0906 190 0212** to find the right solution to your health needs.

Calls cost £1.50 per minute; costs from mobile phones and some other networks may be more. Callers must be aged 18 or over. Lines are open Mon to Fri from 8.30am – 8pm, Sat 8.30am – 6pm.

You can also visit **www.drfoster.co.uk** for information.

Dr Foster Ltd
Sir John Lyon House
5 High Timber Street
London EC4V 3NX

Contents

Acknowledgements

We would like to thank the following individuals and organisations:

Jane Tadman, Arthritis Research Campaign

Dr Madeleine Devey, Arthritis Research Campaign

Emily Butler, Arthritis Care

Daisy O'Clee, CancerBACUP

Claire Boxall, Diabetes UK

Professor Martyn Partridge, Imperial College of Science, Technology and Medicine

National Asthma Campaign

Stroke Association

Foreword by Dr Simon Wallace

Britain is home to many of the world's best doctors. Pick up any of the leading medical journals or attend the major international conferences and you will find many many names from the UK, people who have pioneered new techniques or who are now developing tomorrow's treatments.

Of course we cannot all go to see the country's leading expert when we are affected by illness. And in the overwhelming majority of cases there is no need. However, as the pages of this book show, these people have plenty of very practical advice to patients on how to make sure they are getting looked after properly.

The Dr Foster Good Consultant Guide is designed to give you advice on how to make the most of our health service. We have interviewed some of the leading medical experts in the UK about the advice they give their patients and about the issues that they believe are important in ensuring good quality care in their particular field.

We have selected the doctors largely on the basis of their academic record. These are practising doctors with an exceptional record in publishing new research about the treatment of various illnesses. Of course, that does not mean that these people are therefore better at dealing with patients. But it does mean they have a very good understanding of the area of medicine they are involved in.

One thing is certain. They have some useful tips for everyone – whether it be about the importance of getting the right diagnostic tests, the need to make sure that you are seeing an appropriate doctor, the right questions to ask your doctor before proceeding with treatments or likely trends in new treatments over the coming decade. And there are interesting lessons here for doctors and managers of health services about the ways in which the health services can sometimes fail patients and the areas where steps could be taken to improve services.

The first part of this book distils that advice into the general lessons we can all take with us in dealing with our healthcare needs. The second part looks at the illnesses and conditions that affect most people in this country – asthma, diabetes, arthritis, heart disease, cancer, stroke and Parkinson's disease. In each of these areas we have included interviews with some of the most eminent experts. Finally, at the end of the book, we list those doctors with the strongest record in academic publications over the past six years.

Taken together, this information should help you make sure that you get to see the right doctor and get the best possible treatment.

Dr Simon Wallace
MFPHM DRCOG MBBS

Introduction

Sooner or later most of us will require specialist care in the health service. Under the current UK system, patients are referred to specialists via their general practitioner (GP), whom they rely on heavily for information about the consultant they eventually see.

Whilst GPs often do have a good idea of the interests, strengths and weaknesses of consultants working in local hospitals, it is remarkable how little official information is provided to GPs about the services, interests and standards of specialists and hospitals outside their local area, and it's almost impossible for the patient to get easy access to the basic facts.

With such a dearth of information, finding the best consultant for you can be a hit-and-miss task. How can you be sure you are seeing the right person? What should you look for in a consultant? What should you expect from a consultation? What questions should you ask? How long can you expect to wait? Can you see a specialist outside your area? What are the benefits of specialist centres, compared with general hospitals? This guide answers some of the wealth of questions that most people have when they are faced with the need for specialist care.

You can use the information in this book in conjunction with the Dr Foster website (www.drfoster.co.uk), which not only lists every consultant in the UK by specialty, but also tells you what year they qualified, any special interest they have, the National Health Service (NHS) and private hospitals they work from, and the waiting times at their different clinics. Our website provides the consultants' contact details at their various clinics so that your GP can easily get in touch with them on your behalf. All information in the guides should be used in conjunction with your GP.

Once you have found a consultant who suits your requirements, you will want to find out more about the hospitals they work from and obtain information about any operation you may need to have. Again, by using our website in conjunction with this book, you can compare a consultant's NHS hospital with another nearby. For certain operations, the website tells you which NHS hospitals perform large numbers, which perform few, and which perform them rarely or never.

It also provides you with standardised data on mortality rates in different NHS Trusts for stroke, broken hips and heart bypass surgery.

Not only do we provide you with information on consultants and hospitals, but this book also explains in detail how the system works, what you can expect from it, and how you can get the best out of it.

We give you detailed information on some of the most common, and debilitating, illnesses that patients suffer from in the UK today, including heart disease, Parkinson's disease, arthritis, stroke, diabetes, asthma and cancer. We tell you how the illness is currently treated and what that treatment involves, and we compare how that measures up to treatment in the rest of Europe and the USA. We look at new treatments that are available and tell you whether these are available on the NHS. We examine the training for specialists in each of the above illnesses and tell you what questions you should ask, as well as how to tell the difference between a well-run and a badly run clinic.

In short, by giving you the facts you need in order to be fully informed about your options, Dr Foster enables you to get the best you possibly can out of the health service. No longer will you be kept in the dark about the way in which doctors and hospitals look after your health.

Understanding
the basics

How the system works

What is a consultant?

Consultants are doctors and surgeons with extensive knowledge in a particular area of medicine. They are the most senior grade of specialist and have extensive training in their specialty. Most consultants perform and contribute to medical research, and they often publish academic papers as part of this.

How do I choose a consultant for my condition?

Your GP takes the ultimate decision on which consultant you visit and at which hospital. GPs have extensive knowledge of specialists in the different fields of medicine and are in a good position to choose the best person for you. Once your GP has decided which consultant and hospital is best for you, he or she will refer you. The doctor and hospital will usually be within your local area.

How does my GP decide which consultant is best for me?

GPs will base their decision on their existing knowledge of the consultant and the facilities at the hospital concerned. This knowledge will include feedback from other patients who have seen that consultant, whether the consultant has a special interest in your particular problem and possibly the hospital the consultant works from. You should always ask your GP for his or her reasons for choosing a consultant.

How do I find out more information about the consultant I've been referred to?

Quiz your GP. Ideally you want to see a consultant with a particular interest in your condition, and preferably at a hospital that has a specialist centre in the area of medicine you need treatment in. Ask your GP how experienced the consultant is and whether he or she is interested in the condition you are thought to have. Most GPs have a good overview of the interests of local consultants. You should also ask the hospital for a biography of your consultant. This information is often available in the hospital's prospectus. You can also search the

Dr Foster website to find out information on your consultant (www.drfoster.co.uk). Our website lists consultants by specialty and we give you their areas of expertise, the private and NHS hospitals they work from and the waiting times at their various clinics.

Why is the hospital that I'm referred to important?

It is important you have access to the latest research and treatments for your particular condition. Some hospitals specialise in some conditions more than others and so have doctors with more experience in those areas. For example, a consultant rheumatologist at a specialist centre may deal with 400 cases of lupus each year, whereas a consultant rheumatologist at a local general hospital may only deal with 40 or 50. Specialist centres also have access to new treatments and facilities for research, for the latest tests and for observation. Specialist centres attract leading consultants in that particular specialty and deal with the most complex cases. And if you are having surgery, some hospitals have better outcomes than others.

Can I influence my GP's decision on which consultant or hospital I am referred to?

Your GP is able to refer you to the hospital and consultant of your choice, but there are some limitations. If you express a preference for a hospital or consultant, then so long as your choice is appropriate to the condition for which you are being referred, and it is local, then most GPs will take it into account when referring you. If you are being referred on the NHS, the Primary Care Trust may only fund referrals to local consultants. If your preferred consultant is outside your local area and the Trust refuses to fund your treatment, you should appeal according to the procedures in place at your local Trust.

Can I refer myself to a consultant without seeing my GP first?

No: in the UK you always need to be referred by your GP for both NHS and private referrals. Exceptions to this rule are genitourinary medicine, treatment in the Accident and Emergency department (A&E), if you are admitted to hospital in an emergency, and NHS walk-in centres, providing treatment for minor injuries and illnesses. If you suspect you have a problem that requires specialist attention, go to your GP and discuss it with him or her.

What if my GP won't refer me to a consultant when I want to see one?

Your GP is only obliged to refer you to a consultant if he or she thinks that is appropriate. Your GP does not have to refer you on demand. If you want to see a consultant and your GP won't refer you, ask why. It may be that you have a condition that can be better treated in general practice. If you are unhappy with this decision, change your GP or ask to see another GP in the practice for a second opinion.

I want to go private but my GP still won't refer me to the consultant/hospital of my choice. What can I do?

You do not have a right to be referred privately to a consultant on demand – your GP has to agree that the referral is medically necessary and that the consultant is appropriate. The hospital of your choice may not be equipped to give you the best treatment for your problem. If your GP suggests a different consultant or hospital, ask why. If you are not satisfied with the answer and your GP still won't refer you, then you can either ask to see another doctor in the practice, or change to another practice altogether.

How is a referral made?

Your GP will contact the hospital at which your consultant is based either by letter or by telephone and fax. Non-urgent referrals are usually made by letter and posted to the hospital. Your consultant will read the letter and decide the level of priority, based on its contents. An appointment officer will then allocate an appointment, details of which are sent to you by letter. If your referral is urgent, for example if cancer is suspected, your GP will telephone the hospital to arrange an appointment and will send the referral letter by fax. Often you will be told the date and time of your appointment on that same day.

Do I have a right to see my referral letter?

Yes, and if you feel your GP has not adequately conveyed the pain or discomfort you are experiencing or the effects your condition has on your quality of life, you should ask him or her to rewrite the letter stating these points.

Will I always see the consultant to whom my GP referred me?

There is a high chance you will be seen by a trainee consultant (specialist surgical registrar) or by a nurse consultant, as it is impossible for any consultant to see every patient who has been referred to him or her. However, your consultant will actively supervise your care. Most consultants make a point of seeing the most complicated cases personally.

How long will I have to wait to see a consultant?

There are huge variations between hospitals in waiting times to see a consultant. Your GP's first choice of consultant may have a long waiting list and it may be better to accept the second or third choice rather than wait an unacceptable time. Ask your GP how long the waiting lists are for other consultants available to you. As an outpatient, you should expect to wait no more than 26 weeks. Currently, seven out of ten patients are seen within 13 weeks. As an inpatient, you should expect to wait no longer than 18 months. Currently, three out of four patients are admitted within three months. The Dr Foster website (www.drfoster.co.uk) tells you waiting times at individual hospitals.

How can I tell if I'm waiting longer than normal to see my particular consultant?

Ask your GP to tell you the typical waiting time to see that particular consultant, which will give you an idea of whether you have been waiting longer than normal. All GPs are sent lists of waiting times for consultants in hospitals in their areas and patients are entitled to ask to see these.

Can my GP influence waiting times?

Your GP is able to apply pressure on your behalf, but only if there is a sound and genuine medical reason. If your condition worsens while you are on a waiting list, tell your GP. If you have an urgent problem, you will be given priority over people whose condition is less serious.

What can I do to speed up my waiting time?

Write to the consultant's secretary and say that if there is a cancellation, you are able to accept an appointment at short notice.

You can also ask your GP if there are any other suitable consultants in your area with shorter waiting lists. As a last resort, you can be seen by an NHS consultant privately, who is able to refer you back to the NHS for treatment. The cost of this consultation will be around £200.

What should I do if the appointment I've been given isn't convenient?

Contact the consultant's secretary or the hospital's booking office – the telephone number should be on your appointment card. Explain the situation and they may be able to change the appointment to a date and time that suits you.

What if my appointment is cancelled?

If your appointment is cancelled by the hospital, you should be contacted within seven days with an offer of a new appointment. You should not have an appointment cancelled more than once.

What if I miss my appointment?

It is important that you don't miss your appointment as doing so adds to waiting times. As soon as you realise you have missed your appointment contact the hospital booking office. Some hospitals may tell you that your GP needs to refer you again, others may send you another appointment.

Where will I see my consultant?

You will see your consultant at an outpatient department at the hospital from which he or she works. Outpatient departments are non-ward areas and you will be seen in a private room.

How long will my appointment last?

Outpatient appointments vary in length from seven to 30 minutes, depending on the complexity of the case. After your appointment you can expect to return home.

What if I am unhappy with my GP's choice of consultant after my first visit?

If you are unhappy with the consultant you have been referred to, you should discuss this with your GP. Your GP will be able either to explain why you are not receiving the treatment you expect or, if appropriate, to put your case to the consultant in a constructive way. If you are still unhappy you can ask your GP to refer you to another consultant for a second opinion.

What if my consultant tells me there is nothing wrong but I still feel ill?

Under the Patient's Charter you have the right to be referred for a second opinion if you and your doctor agree that is appropriate. Ask your GP to refer you to another consultant on the NHS, or consider asking for a referral to a private consultant who will be able to see you more quickly.

If I need an operation, how long will I have to wait after my outpatient appointment?

Waiting times vary from one Trust to another and it is impossible to tell how long any one patient will have to wait for an operation. The maximum length of time you will have to wait from seeing the consultant in the outpatient department to being admitted for your operation is 18 months. The average waiting time is three months. You can compare waiting times of hospitals in your area on the Dr Foster website (www.drfoster.co.uk).

Will I get better treatment if I go private?

Most consultants who work in private hospitals also work within the NHS, and therefore the standard of treatment is much the same. However, with private treatment you will bypass NHS waiting lists and your outpatient appointments will last longer and may be more frequent. You will also have the reassurance of knowing that your consultant, rather than a more junior colleague, will perform your operation should you require one. If you are having surgery at a private hospital it is important to find out what facilities a particular hospital has for dealing with serious complications. Not all private hospitals have the range of emergency equipment available at the larger NHS hospitals. As a general rule, a private hospital that draws most of its staff from a major teaching NHS Trust is liable to be a good one.

Can I be a private patient in an NHS hospital?

Many NHS hospitals have facilities for private patients: often either a private wing or single rooms off a main ward. Being a private patient in an NHS hospital may be a good idea if you are having a major operation involving a stay in an intensive care unit as your doctors will have access to NHS equipment and medical staff available around the clock should complications arise.

Can I switch between private and NHS care?

Yes. You can see a consultant privately for assessment and then be referred back to the NHS for surgery, or you can see a consultant on the NHS and then transfer to private care for your operation, should you require one. You can also have diagnostic tests done privately to reduce the time you have to wait for them.

What is private medical insurance?

Private medical insurance is an arrangement whereby, in return for a yearly fee to an insurance company, any private medical treatment you need is paid for by that company. There are many different levels of insurance cover and prices: some schemes only cover the cost of having treatment at named hospitals, whereas others include all aspects of any type of medical care you may need. Insurance premiums increase as people get older and there are often certain restrictions; for example, the cover may exclude treatment for a condition you already have. It is important that you understand what your insurance covers before you take out a policy and before you have any private consultations or treatment.

What are the costs?

The cost of private care varies between hospitals and between consultants. Some private hospitals have a system called 'fixed price care' under which you will be quoted a figure that includes all the likely costs of your stay in hospital. The cost of the operation depends on how long it takes, how complicated it is and how long you're likely to be in hospital afterwards. A heart bypass operation, for example, will probably cost £12,000 or more.

How doctors choose doctors

Patients depend on their GP's knowledge and experience to diagnose their problem, to determine the best treatment, and to suggest the best person to treat it. But what about doctors themselves? They and their families are not immune to illness and disease and at times require access to specialist care, just like everybody else. But unlike everybody else, doctors have contacts and insider knowledge of the system. What is it that doctors look for when they choose another doctor for themselves, a friend or a member of their family?

Sir Donald Irvine, former president of the General Medical Council (GMC), thinks this question is so important that he is planning to conduct research into this very topic on behalf of the King's Fund. 'If doctors go about choosing doctors differently,' he says, 'is there anything we can learn about what it is that they do that we can extend to other people?'

He says that doctors use their intelligence networks to get information when they seek care for themselves and their families. Doctors ask other doctors to recommend experts in a particular field. They then use their knowledge of the system and their networks to obtain information about that specialist's performance as well as the facilities available at a unit and its overall results for a particular procedure, depending on the issues that surround the particular illness.

We asked a range of doctors in different fields what issues they regard as important and what they would look for when seeking care in their areas of medicine for themselves or their families.

Whenever Professor Gianni Angelini, or someone in his family, has a health problem he tries to find out who the best person is in that field. The issues are different for different types of illness, but for heart surgery – Angelini is a leading surgeon at the world-renowned Bristol Heart Institute – he sees the key pieces of information that differentiate the great from the good as being the volume of operations performed, the mortality rate, and the rate of complications, for the unit as well as the surgeon. 'The surgeon, contrary to general belief, is only one member of the team,' Angelini observes. 'If we didn't have a first-class intensive care unit, we would never have had these results.'

The academic position of a unit also contributes to its success, in Angelini's view. 'When you have a very active academic unit, you can take problems, try to find solutions, and then implement those solutions.'

Dr Leonard Shapiro, director of cardiac services at Papworth Hospital in Cambridge, agrees that the number of operations a surgeon carries out would be an important consideration for him if he were being referred to a heart specialist. 'The questions you have to ask your specialist are, "Do you undertake this procedure on a regular basis? How many have you done? Do you specialise solely in this area or is your expertise more general?" For example, in coronary angioplasty, where there are guidelines relating to how many cases should be done by each individual, it would be important to ask, "Do you achieve this number of cases per year?" Evidence suggests that unless you do, you are likely to have less satisfactory outcomes, particularly in the more complex cases.'

But for other diseases, such as lupus, the case isn't so cut and dried. Lupus is a very complex disease, which can attack a number of organs and systems simultaneously, making it difficult to diagnose and treat. For this reason, Dr Graham Hughes, head of the lupus clinic at St Thomas' Hospital in London, thinks that the most important thing is to insist on seeing a specialist with an interest in the condition at a centre that is appropriately set up to manage these complex diseases. Specialist centres, like the one at St Thomas', are becoming more common, but access to one is far from guaranteed for many patients. 'I get many letters from patients whose GP has said, "No, we've got a rheumatologist in this town, you don't need to go to London." I think that is totally wrong,' he says.

Professor Kian Fan Chung, asthma specialist at the Royal Brompton Hospital and the National Heart and Lung Institute, Imperial College, agrees that the hospital context is important: if he was told he needed to see an asthma specialist it is the first thing he would ask about. 'People in general hospitals are often just too busy to have special interests. In many instances, when a patient comes to see you, they haven't had someone sit them down, go through the facts and calm their worries. If you're a general physician and not an expert in the area, you won't be able to provide them with this,' he says.

Seeing a consultant with a special interest in the specific condition, rather than just the general area the condition comes under, is an important consideration for many doctors. Professor John Monson, colorectal cancer specialist at Castle Hill Hospital in Hull, feels that it is advisable to ask about this during the initial consultation. 'If somebody says to me, "Well, you tell me you are a colorectal surgeon, what evidence do you have? Who says you are?" I'm not going to be offended by that question,' he says. 'I think the patient needs to take some responsibility for their own care and not be afraid to ask. If your surgeon is offended by being asked these questions, as a general rule of thumb it's probably not unreasonable to say that you are seeing the wrong person,' he adds.

In the case of Parkinson's disease, too, it is important to find a consultant with a special interest in the condition: misdiagnosis is notoriously common. But Professor Andrew Lees, professor of neurology at the National Hospital for Neurology and Neurosurgery in London, says that if he were recommending a Parkinson's specialist to a colleague, so long as the person were an expert in Parkinson's disease, he would base his decision on the quality of patient care – that is, patience and understanding. 'Good bedside manner is the most important thing,' says Lees. 'Some of the smartest people in medicine have useless bedside skills, and professors generally have a rather bad reputation for that.'

The issues are different again for stroke. While Raymond Tallis, professor of geriatric medicine at the University of Manchester, also agrees that having a special interest in a particular condition is an important consideration, he adds that if he were referred to see a consultant in his field of medicine he would consider specialist training to be crucial too. 'It's not good enough if you have had a stroke to appear under somebody who is just a general physician or a general geriatrician. They have to have had training,' he says. 'Stroke has been an emerging specialty, and what usually happens is that the specialty emerges and then the training comes afterwards. But there is so much to know and to learn that it would be quite unacceptable for anybody to be appointed as a consultant with an interest in stroke without having had proper training on a stroke unit and a commitment to further professional development.'

He adds that although it is the team and teamwork that delivers the gains in any area of medicine, it is important that the team is led by somebody who has had specialist training in that particular area of medicine and who really knows what is what in terms of medical care, the prevention of complications and the driving through and development of protocols for management.

Doctors use their knowledge of medicine and their networks to determine what it is they should look for from a specialist in a specific area of medicine, and then they use their networks to determine the answers to their questions. This being so, it could make a big difference to the quality of healthcare of the population overall if patients had better information on what to look for in a consultant, and information about individual doctors' performance, their specialist interests and the facilities and overall results of the unit they work from. The aim of Dr Foster guides is to extend the intelligence networks of the system into the public domain, giving patients access to knowledge that has traditionally been accessible only to doctors.

What makes a good doctor?

Choosing a doctor is not an easy task because there is no standard procedure you can go by. There is also no definitive list of good doctors and no surefire way to measure exactly what it is that makes a good doctor, although there are markers that patients can look out for. Medical skills and knowledge are critical to being a good doctor, but equally important to patients are communication skills and empathy.

For most people under specialist care, a good doctor is someone who makes them feel better and who treats them with respect and understanding. An effective treatment plan is important in treating disease, but this begins with diagnosis. A good doctor has the experience to diagnose accurately and is also prepared to refer patients on to more specialised colleagues when he or she doesn't have the necessary expert knowledge.

For many diseases, such as Parkinson's, there are no accurate diagnostic tests to confirm the presence of the disease and diagnosis relies on skills and experience. With Parkinson's disease, misdiagnosis occurs because the symptoms of the disease mimic other illnesses; the rate of misdiagnosis can be as high as 51 per cent amongst GPs, compared with 10 per cent for specialist Parkinson's consultants, who have more knowledge and experience of the disease.

Preparedness to pass patients on to experts when they have to is also important for those diseases that have a multitude of symptoms, such as lupus. Lupus can manifest itself in many different ways, and for more complex cases, treatment is best approached by a multi-disciplinary team. A good doctor will be aware of this.

When Ann Shortland was first diagnosed with lupus three years ago by a rheumatologist at the local general hospital to which she had been referred, he immediately referred her on. 'He told me that because of the nature of my condition I needed specialist care by a lupus expert, and he referred me to a specialist centre. I'm very grateful to him for that. I now have continued care from what I believe is one of the best doctors in the country, and that makes me feel very good and very confident,' she says.

For other illnesses, such as heart disease, clinical experience and skill in conducting diagnostic tests and in carrying out surgical procedures are important markers. For instance, the standard test to measure the extent to which arteries are blocked (blocked arteries are the major cause of heart attacks) requires great skill to perform. To ensure that doctors are sufficiently experienced, the Government has suggested that hospitals that do this test should perform at least 500 per year.

Clinical skill also extends to surgery, and for some procedures there are guidelines on how many cases should be done. If a doctor does fewer than a certain number of cases a year the outcomes are much less satisfactory than for surgeons who do more than that number. Key pieces of information that differentiate the great from the good for surgery include the volume of operations performed, the mortality rate and the rate of complications – this applies to the unit as well as the surgeon. Good doctors work as part of a team, and have access to quality equipment should complications arise.

The main problem in identifying a good doctor is gaining access to information on their success or failures. Whilst some hospitals openly publish mortality figures for individual surgeons performing specific operations, this is far from the norm and most of the country remains largely in the dark about surgical performance. Even GPs often don't have access to information about local performance indicators. But following high-profile scandals, this is beginning to change. The Bristol hospital at the centre of the scandal involving the deaths of babies undergoing heart surgery now publishes on the internet the mortality rate of its surgeons. However, it is important to remember that even the best doctors have failures. Mortality rates alone are not enough to determine who the best doctors are.

The inquiry that followed the Bristol scandal looked at the issue of what makes a good doctor and the general conclusion was that, as well as intellectual and academic competence, doctors require good interpersonal skills and positive attitudes towards patients and colleagues.

According to the inquiry panel, there is evidence of a link between good communication and positive outcomes for patients, and that poor communication and failure of teamwork can lead to errors. Communication means talking to patients and explaining the condition they have, going through all the treatment options available, and spelling out the short- and long-term prognoses. If a patient requires surgery, communication means explaining the operation, and telling the patient what the risks are and what to expect when going into hospital, while in hospital and when he or she goes home.

But the British public feels let down in the communication stakes. According to a recent study published in the *British Medical Journal* (*BMJ*), the biggest complaint among patients in Britain is that doctors tend to take too little account of their feelings. Patients want to be treated like a person, not just another case. They want doctors who listen to them and who explain medical procedures in a clear and simple way.

Gianni Angelini, leading heart surgeon and head of the Bristol Heart Institute, feels that the ability to communicate is the only thing that can convince a patient that the consultant is doing everything possible. 'If you can communicate with people, tell them honestly what's going on, they will never complain. This is my personal experience. It's when you try to hide things, or not interact, that people get suspicious and then you get into trouble,' he says.

Communication skills should be honed at medical school, but the selection criteria for medical students do not take account of these wider issues. Instead, emphasis is placed on academic ability, and there are claims of discrimination against working-class and ethnic minority applicants. In a discussion paper, however, the British Medical Association (BMA) board of medical education argues that there is no good evidence to suggest that the selection for medical schools 'has been inappropriate in terms of the quality of the doctors produced'.

The BMA does perhaps have a point. The *BMJ* study shows that British doctors top the polls as the most trustworthy and hardworking of all professionals. In 2000, trust in doctors rose two points on the previous year, to 89 per cent, and overall satisfaction dropped just one point, to 89 per cent, despite the unprecedented number of medical scandals and transgressions in recent years.

Making the most of your care

Learn as much as you can about your condition before you meet your consultant.

The more you learn about your condition, the more questions you will have, so it is helpful to do some research before you meet your consultant. Start by looking on the internet or at your local library. Your GP can put you in touch with support groups for specific conditions, and these can also be a good source of information. Part 2 of this guide lists support groups that you may find helpful.

Make sure that you are seeing the best consultant for you.

Question your GP thoroughly about why they chose that particular consultant for you. Make sure that your consultant has a special interest in your condition and, if not, ask to be referred to one who does. If you are being referred on the NHS, the Primary Care Trust may only fund referrals to local consultants. If your preferred consultant is outside your local area and the Trust refuses to fund your treatment, you should appeal according to the procedures in place at your local Trust.

Ask about the hospital as well as the consultant. It is preferable to be treated at a hospital with a specialist centre in the area of medicine that you need care in, rather than at a general hospital. Consultants in general hospitals may be dealing with a wide range of diagnoses rather than areas of special interest; for example, in the area of orthopaedics you may see a general orthopaedic surgeon rather than an orthopaedic surgeon who has specialised in hand surgery. Specialist centres also have greater access to new treatments, as well as better facilities for tests and research.

If your GP won't share information with you about specialist consultants, do some research. Patient support groups and the internet are both great sources of information. Alternatively, you can search the Dr Foster website (www.drfoster.co.uk), which publishes lists of consultants and their specialties.

Write down the questions you want to ask before your first appointment.

It is important to write down a list of questions about your condition or anything else that worries you and to take it with you when you see your consultant. Questions may include:

- Do I really have the disease my doctor thinks I have?
- What disease do you think I have?
- Can you explain that condition to me?
- What treatments are available?
- Which is the best treatment for me?
- What can I expect to get from the treatment?
- When is it going to work?
- How long am I going to be on it?
- Are there any side-effects?
- What is the short-term prognosis?
- What is the long-term prognosis?

Make sure you understand what your consultant says.

It is vital that you understand what the consultant says to you; if you don't follow what he or she is saying, calmly insist on having your condition explained further, and in plain English. If you are confused, say so and ask your consultant to slow down. Take notes during your appointment so you don't forget what you are told, or take a friend or relative with you who can take notes on your behalf. At the end of your appointment make sure your consultant has given you a treatment plan and that you understand any follow-up procedures you may need to have. Ask your consultant when you will next see him or her again. If you have any questions in the meantime, write them down and raise them at your next consultation.

If you need an operation, ask questions.

It is important that you are fully informed not only about any procedure you are to undergo, but also about the experience of the consultant conducting the operation and the results of the unit in that particular procedure. Your consultant should be able to answer all relevant questions, which may include:

- Who is going to carry out the operation?
- How many times has the surgeon carried out this procedure?

- What is the mortality rate of the surgeon?
- What is the rate of complications for the surgeon?
- How many of these operations does the unit do in total?
- What is the mortality rate of the unit?
- What is the rate of complications for the unit?
- What are the benefits of the operation compared with not having it done?
- What are the risks involved and what can be done to minimise these?
- Are there any alternatives to surgery?
- How long is the expected recovery time?

Insist that your consultant answers your questions.
You have a right as a patient to be fully informed about any procedure you are to undertake, and your consultant has a duty to answer any questions you have. If your consultant is unhappy about answering any of your questions, raise this with your GP and ask him or her to speak on your behalf. If you are seeing a more junior specialist, then ask to speak to the consultant. As a last resort, discuss with your GP the option of being referred to another consultant.

If you need surgery, your consultant may not carry it out.
Your consultant is only one member of a team. Your consultant is responsible for managing your care, assisted by a team of doctors. While you may see your consultant at hospital appointments and on the ward, there is no certainty that he or she will perform your operation. There are several grades of surgeon with different levels of experience who work under the direction of the consultant. Always ask your consultant who will perform your operation and how much experience that surgeon has had.

Be prepared with a list of questions before you meet your surgeon prior to your operation.
Your surgeon will always meet with you before the operation. You should use this opportunity to ask more questions about the immediate physical effects of the operation. Have a list of questions written down, the answers to which should be provided in plain English. If you don't understand anything, ask again.

Questions might include:

- What will be done if complications arise during surgery?
- Where will I be cut and how big is the scar likely to be?
- How soon can I get up after the operation?
- When will I be able to start eating and drinking?
- What pain relief am I likely to need and will I have to ask for it?
- Will I have any drips, drains or catheters and if so, what for?
- How long will I be in hospital?
- When can I start driving again?
- When can I go back to work?
- When can I resume playing sport?
- Will I need to attend the outpatient clinic afterwards?

Knowing how the system works, what you can expect from it and how to get the best out of it can make a real difference to getting better or to living better with a debilitating condition. But being fully informed also means being armed with the clinical detail and expert opinion about your condition. We've asked some of the UK's leading doctors working in heart disease, Parkinson's disease, arthritis, stroke, diabetes, asthma and cancer what they think is important for you to know about managing your illness. In the second part of this guide, we've drawn on their expert opinion to take you through these common conditions, explaining what they are, how they are currently treated and how that compares to treatment in the rest of Europe and the USA. We look at new treatments that are available and tell you whether these are available on the NHS or whether you might be better off being treated privately. We examine the training for specialists in each of the above illnesses and tell you what questions you should ask, as well as how to tell the difference between a well-run and a badly run clinic. And if you need to know more, we tell you how to get in touch with patient groups and the specialists featured in this guide. One message comes through strongly from all of them: being well informed is good for your health.

Specialties
and specialists

Arthritis and related disorders

What is the specialty?

Rheumatology, rheumatology and general medicine, rheumatology and rehabilitation and/or orthopaedics, paediatric rheumatology.

What is arthritis and how many people are affected?

Arthritis is the overall term for a number of different conditions – over 200 in all – in which the joints become swollen and painful. It includes osteoarthritis, inflammatory arthritis, lupus and gout. It's estimated that seven million adults in the UK (15 per cent of the population) have long-term health problems caused by arthritis, and almost nine million have visited their GP in the past year with arthritis and related conditions. Osteoarthritis (OA), the most common form, affects as many as 10 to 20 per cent of people aged over 64, and is on the increase. It is the most common single cause of arthritis-linked disability. Inflammatory arthritic conditions such as rheumatoid arthritis (RA), juvenile idiopathic arthritis, psoriatic arthritis and ankylosing spondylitis affect around one in fifty people. Rheumatoid arthritis is the most common form of inflammatory arthritis, affecting around one in a hundred people – over 420,000 people in England and Wales and 15,000 of these severely. Nine out of ten people with aggressive forms of this disease will become clinically disabled within 20 years.

How is it currently treated?

In the past, people with arthritis became steadily more disabled and faced an early death. In the twentieth century, gold and aspirin, both of which are still used today as treatments for rheumatoid arthritis, began to be used. However, the big breakthrough came in 1948 with the discovery of steroids by Philip Hench. The discovery that brought Hench the Nobel Prize transformed life for thousands of sufferers. Unfortunately, the side-effects of large doses of steroids meant that many people continued to die early. The next big steps forward were the development of non-steroidal anti-inflammatory drugs (NSAIDs), which still form one of the mainstays of treatment, and more recently of a sophisticated type of NSAID called COX-2, which is said to avoid the gastro-intestinal side-effects of older NSAIDs.

Current treatment will depend on the type of arthritis you have. Infective arthritis is likely to need a course of antibiotics. If you have gout, you will be prescribed treatments to prevent further attacks such as allopurinol, probenecid and sulphinpyrazone. Many types of arthritis will be treated with painkillers and/or anti-inflammatory drugs, either aspirin-based or more often one of the many NSAIDs on the market. Chronic, progressive forms of arthritis such as rheumatoid arthritis, lupus and psoriatic arthritis often need stronger medications such as corticosteroids and/or immunosuppressive drugs. If these do not work or stop working, the doctor may move on to the newer drugs (see p.32).

OSTEOARTHRITIS

Osteoarthritis can affect all joints of the body, but is usually found in the fingers, knees, hips and spine. The process begins with cartilage becoming thin and uneven, and eventually it can wear out completely. At the same time, the joint capsule becomes thicker, and more synovial (lubricating) fluid is manufactured which makes the joint swell. In addition to cartilage degeneration, bony spurs grow, causing inflammation in the surrounding tissues.

Treatment is aimed at alleviating pain and improving mobility. It may include:

- **Exercise:** to keep your joints mobile and strengthen muscles that support the joints.
- **Medications to control pain:** including painkillers such as paracetamol, aspirin and, less often, NSAIDs. Sometimes injections of corticosteroids are helpful.
- **Physiotherapy:** for example, heat or cold treatment, ultrasound, hydrotherapy to help ease pain.
- **Splints and other aids:** for example, walking stick to alleviate stress on the joints and prevent further strain.
- **Weight management (diet and exercise):** to prevent extra stress on the joints.
- **Surgery (see p.30):** if the condition is seriously affecting your everyday activities.

RHEUMATOID ARTHRITIS

Rheumatoid arthritis can be a very aggressive inflammatory condition, affecting fingers, thumbs, wrists, knees and feet. It may involve many other areas of the body and make you generally unwell. The severity of attacks is extremely variable, and ranges from a single episode to severe disabling illness.

The aim of treatment is to alleviate pain and to reduce inflammation in order to minimise damage to your joints. Early treatment is essential in order to prevent further damage to the joints. A huge number of medications are available. They include:

- **Non-steroidal anti-inflammatory drugs (NSAIDs):** for example, aspirin, indomethacin, naproxen, ibuprofen, piroxicam, diclofenac, meloxicam, nabumetone. Less popular today than in the past, ibuprofen is available over the counter, but other NSAIDS require a prescription. NSAIDs do nothing to slow the progress of disease in rheumatoid arthritis. Their biggest problem is that they can irritate the stomach and lead to the development of gastric and duodenal ulcers.

- **COX-2 inhibitors:** for example, rofecoxib, celecoxib. These suppress the activity of an enzyme called cyclo-oxygenase (COX) that is involved in inflammation and pain. The drugs are highly effective in quelling inflammation and when they first came on to the market were hailed as a great step forward in terms of causing fewer gastro-intestinal side-effects. Unfortunately, the most recent research has found that they may not be so gastro-protective as originally thought when used over the long term.

- **Corticosteroids (steroids or glucocorticoids):** for example, cortisone, prednisolone. These are synthetic versions of the body's own natural cortisone hormones. They work by preventing the body from manufacturing inflammatory chemicals and by reducing the activity of the immune system, which is responsible for sparking off attacks of rheumatoid arthritis. They can be given in tablet form or by injection into an inflamed joint.

- **Disease-modifying anti-rheumatic drugs (DMARDs):** for example, gold by injection or tablets, D-penicillamine, sulphasalazine, methotrexate, azathioprine, cyclophosphamide, ciclosporin, anti-malarial drugs, leflunomide. Slow-acting drugs are used to quell inflammation. Although in the past DMARDs were usually used only for people with X-ray signs of joint erosion, today they are used earlier and more intensively in order to try to slow progression of the disease and so spare the joints from permanent, irreversible damage. They are often prescribed in combinations of two and sometimes three different drugs as it has been found that these control disease activity better than prescribing them singly. In the UK, sulphasalazine is the most popular DMARD, with eight out of ten people with rheumatoid arthritis having it prescribed in the first year, followed usually by methotrexate.

- **Biological agents:** for example, etanercept and inflixamib. These relatively new treatments consist of genetically engineered proteins that are part of the immune system. Etanercept and inflixamib are both anti-TNF alpha drugs, which work by switching off tumour necrosis factor (TNF), a chemical that stimulates cells to produce the inflammatory response that leads to swelling of the joints.

SURGERY AND SURGICAL PROCEDURES

A number of operations and other surgical procedures may be performed if the joints are badly damaged and cannot be helped by other treatments.

- **Arthroplasty (partial or total joint replacement).** The most common joints to be replaced are the hips and knees, although the shoulders and elbows (occasionally the knuckles – metacarpal phalangeal joints) can also be replaced. The surgeon removes part or all of the damaged joint and replaces it. Joint implants are made of metal or plastic materials. Traditionally, surgeons used a special cement to fix the artificial joint to the bones. The biggest problem is that the cement may crack after several years, causing the implant to become unstable and requiring further surgery. Researchers are looking at new ways of manufacturing and applying cement. Newer cementless replacement joints are also available, which have a porous surface, allowing those with good bone quality to form a strong attachment.
- **Arthrodesis (joint fusion).** This is done to ease pain and improve stability in the spine, wrist, ankle or foot. The surgeon removes the cartilage and a thin layer of bone from the ends of the two

bones to be fused and joins the two ends. As fresh bone cells grow, the two bones fuse together. Pins, rods or plates may be used to keep the bones in place.

- **Arthroscopic debridement.** The surgeon sucks out loose fragments of bone, cartilage or synovium (the membrane coating joint capsules) that are the source of joint pain, using an instrument called an arthroscope to view the joint. Most often used for osteoarthritis.

- **Synovectomy.** An operation to remove inflamed synovial tissue in order to reduce pain and swelling and delay or even prevent destruction of the cartilage. Used for fingers, wrists and knees.

- **Osteotomy.** An operation in which the surgeon cuts and repositions the bones in order to correct deformities.

How does that measure up to treatment in the rest of Europe and the USA?

Although treatment is broadly similar to that of the UK, some of the newer treatments, such as the new anti-TNF drugs (see p.32), which have only just been licensed in the UK, are much more widely used in the rest of Europe. The Prosorba therapy (see p.32) will soon be available in certain European countries, such as Germany and France, although not all rheumatologists are convinced of its effectiveness. Glucosamine sulphate, a nutritional supplement, which has been shown in several trials to be effective in relieving pain in osteoarthritis (although some rheumatologists are sceptical), is more widely used in Europe, especially in Germany.

Where the UK does differ significantly from the rest of Europe is in the number of specialists. A survey by the Arthritis and Rheumatism Council Epidemiology Research Unit in 1993 found that only two European countries – the Irish Republic and Portugal – had fewer rheumatologists per 100,000 of the population than the UK (although these figures may be a little misleading since, for example, in Germany there are a number of 'spa doctors' who are regarded locally as rheumatologists but have not had any formal training). The British Society for Rheumatology recommends that there should be one rheumatologist per 80,000 people, but according to Arthritis Care, in many areas this is likely to be insufficient.

A whole host of new arthritis therapies have appeared on the USA market, some of which are beginning to become available in the UK. They include new COX-2 inhibitors, anti-TNF drugs, Prosorba therapy (see below), and two viscosupplements (see below) (see Isaacs, p.45–7; Isenberg, p.48).

What new treatments are available?

- **New DMARDs.** A number of new DMARDs are becoming available. The first of these, leflunomide (Arava), is already on the market. It may be prescribed in combination with methotrexate if methotrexate alone is ineffective.
- **Biological treatments.** These include anti-TNF drugs such as etanercept (Enbrel) and inflixamib (Remicade), recently approved by the National Institute for Clinical Excellence (NICE), and a number of other agents that act on the body's immune system.
- **Viscosupplements.** For example, hyaluronan, hylan G-F20. These are synthetic fluids that mimic the synovial fluid that lubricates the joints, used to relieve the pain of knee osteoarthritis. They are administered by a short series of injections and in a few cases can bring pain relief for six to thirteen months.
- **Prosorba therapy (protein-A immunoadsorption).** A procedure for people with severe rheumatoid arthritis that has not responded to DMARDs. Not a drug at all, but a procedure that involves drawing blood from your arm, separating plasma from red blood cells and treating it through a cylinder the size of a tin of tomatoes containing a sand-like substance coated with protein A, a molecule that binds antibodies. The treated plasma is then remixed with the red blood cells and injected back into the body. Treatment involves 12 weekly sessions of around two to two- and -a- half hours. Side-effects include fatigue and flu-like symptoms. It can take 12 to 16 weeks to work, but early reports suggest it can bring remission for up to a year and a half in people with recalcitrant rheumatoid arthritis.

Can I get these on the NHS?

In 2001, two anti-TNF drugs, etanercept and infliximab, were approved by NICE, and others are in the pipeline. However, they can cost as much as £8,000–9,500 a year, and are currently licensed only to be prescribed for people with severe rheumatoid arthritis who have failed to respond to two or three DMARDs. Although they have been approved, there are some concerns that because of their expense, doctors may be reluctant to prescribe them.

What treatments are in the pipeline?

A number of other biological treatments are likely to be on the market in the not too distant future. One of these, Kineret (anakinra), which is already available in the USA, works by blocking an immune system chemical called interleukin 1. Another more drastic treatment is stem cell transplantation. Stem cells are the primitive cells that are capable of developing into any cell in the body. The treatment involves giving a dose of an immunosuppressive drug plus a daily injection to stimulate the growth of stem cells and move them from the bone marrow to the blood. A week later, the cells are 'harvested' (collected from the blood) and frozen. Six weeks later, you are taken into hospital and given a large dose of immunosuppressive drug to destroy the bone marrow cells and knock out the immune system. The stem cells are defrosted and the immune system is regenerated. At present, the technique is still only experimental. Further trials are needed, and so far only a handful of patients have had the treatment, but it could prove promising for people with severe rheumatoid arthritis.

Another experimental treatment that is available in the UK is the antibody to CD2O (rituximab) which marks B lymphocytes, helping drugs to find infected cells and kill them. Encouraging open studies have been followed by a multi-centre trial now in progress.

As far as osteoarthritis is concerned, researchers are looking at autologous chondrocyte implantation (ACI) or articular cartilage transplantation (ACT), a technique that involves extracting the healthy cells that form cartilage via arthroscopy. These are then cultured in the lab before being injected back into the joint. The technique is intended for younger people with damaged or defective cartilage. At present it is on offer in only a handful of specialist orthopaedic centres in the UK. NICE evaluated the procedure in 2000 but didn't recommend it for routine treatment.

A further pioneering treatment is a new form of immunotherapy against lupus. In this technique, patients are injected with antibodies that specifically target the B-cells of the immune system, causing them to be destroyed. B-cells are at the centre of the mechanism by which lupus damages the body, so if you can stop the B-cells in their tracks, then this might stop the disease (Isenberg, p.48).

Who treats it?

In the first instance you should see your GP, who may be able to diagnose you. Most people with osteoarthritis are diagnosed and treated by their GPs. However, experts say that people who suspect they have osteoarthritis should see a rheumatologist in order to get a proper diagnosis.

If you have one of the chronic inflammatory types of arthritis, such as rheumatoid arthritis, you should definitely see a consultant rheumatologist as early as possible in the course of your disease, as it is important to start treatment early. There's also a small handful of paediatric rheumatologists for children with juvenile arthritis (see Woo, p.53–5). If you need surgery, the rheumatologist should refer you to an orthopaedic surgeon.

What training will the specialist have?

Before becoming a consultant, your doctor will have had a general medical training, which includes five years at university followed by one year as a House Officer, before gaining registration with the General Medical Council. They will then have spent two to three years as a Senior House Officer in various medical disciplines. This is followed by a five- or six-year period of specialist registrar training, working in different hospitals, leading to a Certificate of Completion of Specialist Training that is recognised throughout Europe. In the fifth year and post-certification, doctors are encouraged to train to become sub-specialists.

Compared with other medical specialties, rheumatology is a relatively new discipline that really began only in the 1950s. For a specialist rheumatologist, their registrar training will have been in rheumatology or general medicine. Because rheumatoid arthritis is an autoimmune disease, many of those who specialise in rheumatology do so because of an interest in immunology. Paediatric rheumatologists will have trained in paediatrics followed by additional training in rheumatology.

Where will I receive care?

Most of your care will take place in the outpatient department at a specialist arthritis or rheumatology clinic. Occasionally you may need admission to hospital, although the number of rheumatology beds is fairly limited and you may end up being cared for on a general medical ward.

What questions should I ask about my treatment?
Medication

- What treatment plan are you proposing?
- What drug(s) (e.g. NSAIDs, DMARDs, steroids) will be prescribed?
- Will I be prescribed more than one drug?
- How often will I have to take them?
- How will they be delivered – pill form, injection?
- How long will it take before I experience an improvement in my symptoms?
- What side-effects can I expect?
- How will I be monitored (e.g. chest X-ray, liver and kidney function tests)?
- Are there any contraindications (e.g. pregnancy, breastfeeding)?
- Can I drink alcohol while taking this drug?
- Are there likely to be any other drug interactions (including over-the-counter, herbal and nutritional supplements)?
- Can I have immunisations while taking this drug? (People taking etanercept, for example, should avoid live vaccines such as polio, rubella and yellow fever.)
- What will happen if I do get side-effects?
- Are there any other drugs you can prescribe?
- How should I manage flare-ups?
- What if the drugs I am taking stop working?
- How often do I need to visit the clinic?
- Is there anything I can do to help myself?
- Can diet help control symptoms?
- What exercise is it safe to take?
- Is there a physiotherapy pool I can use?
- Can you refer me to a specialist pain clinic?

Joint replacement

- Will I be able to have a joint replacement?
- Are there any age limits?
- What exactly does the procedure involve?
- What are the benefits and risks?
- What materials (e.g. metal or plastic) will be used for the joint replacement?
- Will cement be used?
- If anything goes wrong what can be done to put it right?
- How long will I have to stay in hospital?
- How long will it take me to recover so that I can do normal activities?
- How long has this procedure been in use?
- Who will do the operation?
- How many operations of this type have you done?
- What is the success rate for this type of operation?
- How long can I expect the joint to last?
- Are there any alternative treatments?

What will my treatment involve?

Osteoarthritis

You will usually be cared for by your GP, unless the disease becomes severe. Treatment will be at home and may involve outpatient physiotherapy and/or pain management. Arthritis Care (see p.41) have pioneered patient empowerment groups designed to help you think more positively about your condition and manage pain. You may need to be admitted to hospital if you need a joint replacement or one of the surgical procedures outlined above.

Rheumatoid arthritis

In the past decade, doctors have come to appreciate that for many patients rheumatoid arthritis is best treated aggressively in the early stages to prevent joint destruction. Making an early diagnosis requires a battery of tests and a specialist doctor. Although rapid access clinics are the ideal, in most parts of the UK patients must join the standard NHS waiting lists for these (see Isaacs, p.45–7).

One of the most popular current approaches is known as the 'saw tooth' strategy. Research suggests that this strategy can result in a remission rate of around 30 per cent. The approach involves using a combination of DMARDs continuously right from the start. You are then seen at regular intervals by the specialist and treatment goals will be established in terms of a reduction of disease activity and how disabling the disease is. The specialist should modify your treatment as and when necessary, adding in steroids or other DMARDs if the strategy does not bring an appreciable diminishment of disease activity. Painkilling drugs and NSAIDs should be used as an adjunct to help relieve symptoms.

Another approach, the 'step down' approach, involves attacking the disease with a combination of DMARDs in order to send it into remission. As the disease remits, the stronger, more toxic medications are gradually withdrawn. The aim is to keep the disease under control while limiting the number of toxic drugs you have to take. Steroid drugs and NSAIDs will be used to control symptoms while the DMARDs take effect.

All the drugs used to treat rheumatoid arthritis and some of those used to treat osteoarthritis cause side-effects. Gastro-intestinal problems are a common side-effect of NSAIDs, and recent research suggests that there is also an increased risk of heart failure in people taking the drugs.

Most people with arthritis will need to be admitted to hospital at some time during the course of their illness, for example, for corrective surgery, to help straighten out deformed hands.

What makes a REAL difference to getting better?
Doctors prefer to talk in terms of controlling arthritis rather than getting better. But there are a number of factors that can make a difference.
- **Seeing the right specialist.** Arthritis organisations are concerned that too many people don't get to see a rheumatologist, but are treated by their GPs or sent inappropriately to see an orthopaedic surgeon. In some areas (for example, Stoke-on-Trent) there are GP/rheumatologists. In others, there are outreach teams. However, in most areas you will need to be referred to an arthritis clinic at your local hospital.
- **Early treatment.** In the case of rheumatoid arthritis in particular, early treatment with DMARDs is crucial to controlling the disease and reducing joint damage.

- **An accessible, multi-disciplinary team.** This should consist of a specialist rheumatologist, specialist arthritis nurses, physiotherapists, occupational therapists who may visit you at home to assess your lifestyle and advise on any modifications (such as special taps or raised chairs to help ease the burden of arthritis on your daily life) and other healthcare professionals, such as an orthotist (applicance fitter), who can help fit and supply splints and appliances, a podiatrist to advise on footcare and recommend inserts to go in your shoes, and social workers who can help you apply for any benefits such as disability allowance. You may also see a dietitian, for example, if you are losing weight, or a psychologist.
- **The availability of a specialist arthritis nurse.** Research carried out by the Arthritis Research Campaign suggests that patients with arthritis do better in clinics run by senior nurses than those run by junior doctors. The results are attributed to the fact that nurses look at the person holistically, taking into account the effect of the disease on all aspects of his or her life.
- **Self-management.** Learning to live with your arthritis and to manage pain are important elements in controlling the disease. Self-management can include exercise, diet and positive thinking. Arthritis Care (see p.41) runs patient empowerment courses.

What is the difference between a well-run and a badly run clinic?

According to the Arthritis Research Campaign and Arthritis Care, the features of a well-run arthritis clinic include:

Early referral

The clinic should have enough rheumatologists and a multi-disciplinary team to make sure that you are seen soon after referral to the hospital by your GP.

Easy access

The clinic should be easily accessible, with features such as automatic doors, ramps, raised chairs and assistance for people with wheelchairs if facilities are any distance from the entrance.

Minimal waiting times

Waiting times should not be lengthy. Block booking (booking several people for the appointment slot) should not happen.

Time to talk

Because arthritis can affect every aspect of your life, it is important that you have enough time at the appointment to discuss all your concerns.

Flexible consultation

The course of arthritis, especially rheumatoid arthritis, can be extremely variable, with sudden, severe flare-ups. It's important that you should be able to call or drop in to see the arthritis nurse and be able to be referred to the doctor quickly if necessary.

Combined clinics

If surgery is recommended, you should be able to attend a combined clinic, where you can see a specialist rheumatologist and orthopaedic surgeon, and other health professionals such as a physiotherapist and occupational therapist if necessary.

Car parking and transport

There should be enough Orange Badge parking spaces for people with arthritis and arrangements for transport to and from hospital for those with flare-ups who can't get to the hospital under their own steam.

Will I get better treatment if I go privately?

In 2001, there were 62,000 people waiting for hip or knee replacement operations. Going privately may mean you see a specialist more quickly, although the treatment should be broadly the same as you would receive on the NHS. Going privately may also give you access to some of the newer treatments that may be limited by cash constraints on the NHS.

Will I get better treatment if I go abroad?

In July 2000, the European Court of Justice ruled that patients waiting an undue length of time on the NHS had a right to seek treatment elsewhere in the EU and be paid for by the NHS. The first pilot projects, which took place in early 2002, involved patients from Kent and the south-east travelling to France, and included several needing hip and knee replacements.

Knee replacements cost on average £4,400 (NHS), £8,500 (private) and £3,000 (France); hip replacements £3,900 (NHS), £7,600 (private) and £4,000 (France).

What support will I be offered by the clinic and are there any independent support groups I can join?

A good arthritis clinic should provide back-up support from a range of different healthcare professionals (see p.38). In particular, you should be able to see an arthritis nurse to talk about the various treatment options, and receive a full range of information leaflets about different drugs and specific treatments, as well as benefits information and details of the self-help groups and any self-management programmes in your area, such as Arthritis Care's Challenging Arthritis. The best clinics may offer drop-in consultation (see p.39) and a telephone helpline that you or your GP or other care professionals can use to get advice as and when it is needed.

Useful addresses

Arthritis Care
18 Stephenson Way
London NW1 2HD
Tel 020 7380 6500 (10 am to 4 pm Monday to Friday)
Helpline 080 8800 4050 (12 noon to 4 pm Monday to Friday)
www.arthritiscare.org.uk

Arthritis Research Campaign
Copeman House
St Mary's Court, St Mary's Gate
Chesterfield
Derbyshire S41 7TD
Tel 0870 850 5000
www.arc.org.uk

The Children's Chronic Arthritis Association
Ground Floor, Amber Gate
City Wall Road
Worcester WR1 2AH
Tel 01905 745595
www.ccaa.org.uk/

Lupus UK
1 Eastern Road
Romford
Essex RM1 3NH
Tel 01708 731251

National Rheumatoid Arthritis Society
Briarwood House, 11 College Avenue
Maidenhead
Berkshire SL6 6AR
Tel 01628 670606
www.rheumatoid.org.uk

Expert opinions

Dr Graham Hughes

Rheumatoid arthritis is part of a family of illnesses known as autoimmune diseases, in which the patient's own immune system starts to attack the body tissue. The group also includes a number of less well-known disorders. Dr Graham Hughes is head of the lupus clinic at St Thomas' Hospital in London, which specialises in treating patients with three of these – lupus, Hughes syndrome and vasculitis.

Hughes' work has had dramatic results for many of his patients. In 1983, he identified a previously unrecognised condition – Hughes syndrome – and subsequently he has played a major part in developing effective treatments for it.

In the past, women who suffered from this unknown and incurable disorder had only a 20 per cent chance of having a successful pregnancy. At the St Thomas' unit, with modern treatments this has risen to almost 90 per cent. More recently, it has been shown that the condition may be responsible for as many as one in five strokes in younger people.

One of his biggest concerns is that people with these less well-known conditions do not get to see a specialist. Specialist centres like the one at St Thomas' are becoming more common, but access to one is far from guaranteed for many patients. 'I get many letters from patients whose GP has said, "No, we've got a rheumatologist in this town, you don't need to go to London." I think that is totally wrong.'

It is important to see an expert because the conditions treated at the clinic can attack a number of organs and systems simultaneously, making them particularly difficult to diagnose and treat. 'These are some of the sickest patients coming to St Thomas',' says Hughes, 'But you can treat them. We now see what used to be thought of as a dread disease as being totally treatable. Patients can come off all their medicines and live a normal life.'

A multi-system disease requires input from many different medical specialties, and the St Thomas' unit is configured to provide this. 'We don't do general rheumatology here,' says Hughes. 'The reason is that these diseases are so complex; we think you need a special unit. Instead of just seeing a rheumatologist, or a dermatologist if you have got a skin problem, we have got a kidney doctor who comes here, a haematologist who looks after blood clotting, and even a lupus pregnancy clinic with obstetrics doctors once a week. It's really becoming more specialised.'

It was Hughes' work with lupus patients that led to his discovery of Hughes syndrome. 'I reported a group of patients from the lupus clinic who had a tendency to blood clotting,' he says. 'It would clot anywhere in the body. But we found there was one blood test that could pick out this risk. It's called an anticardiolipin antibody test – a very long-winded name, but it's a simple blood test.'

Patients whose blood tests positive for the condition are at increased risk of blood clots, and the organs at greatest risk are the brain and, in pregnant women, the placenta. 'If a pregnant woman has these antibodies, the placenta can get clotted up. The baby does not get blood, it withers and there is a miscarriage. Some of these women have 10 or 12 miscarriages. The exciting thing now is that if a woman has a miscarriage and a positive blood test, they can be treated and have a successful pregnancy.' With treatment, the chances of a woman with Hughes syndrome having a successful pregnancy have increased from under 20 per cent to almost 90 per cent.

'In the brain, it's even more interesting,' says Hughes. 'Patients can get migraines or severe headaches, or it can be something more sinister such as mini-strokes. If you look at strokes in people aged 45 or under, one in five are due to Hughes syndrome. That's phenomenally important economically to the country.'

'Other patients don't get strokes, but they get memory loss or speech problems. They think they are getting Alzheimer's. Some of them get pins and needles and balance problems, and are wrongly diagnosed as having multiple sclerosis. The minute you start to treat them it clears up. It's like a fog lifting.'

Strokes, miscarriages and other blood clotting problems such as deep vein thrombosis (DVT) contribute considerably to the workload of hospitals all over the country, and studies are currently being carried out into the proportion of these events that are linked to Hughes syndrome.

For patients labelled with Hughes syndrome or lupus, Hughes' first piece of advice is to get some literature about the condition. National patient support groups such as Lupus UK and the Hughes Syndrome Foundation (www.hughes-syndrome.org) publish information in booklets and on the internet, and can put patients in touch with other sufferers in their local area. 'I think drawing up a list of questions is worthwhile too,' he says, 'Because it's absolutely standard to go out of the clinic and think, "I forgot to ask."'

However, the most important thing is to insist on seeing a specialist with an interest in the condition at a centre that is appropriately set up to manage these complex diseases.

Professor John Isaacs

An innovative clinic in Leeds is giving patients with early signs of rheumatoid arthritis an improved chance of slowing the progress of this crippling condition in its early stages, says Professor John Isaacs, reflecting on his time as a consultant rheumatologist at the centre (he is newly appointed to the Freeman Hospital, Newcastle).

Rheumatoid arthritis is a chronic condition that can make a healthy person irreversibly disabled in just a few months. It is also a difficult disease to diagnose, because many people who come to their GPs with joint pain actually have other, more benign forms of arthritis that clear up in a relatively short time. 'The important question is deciding which patients with joint symptoms are going to develop rheumatoid arthritis, as opposed to the self-limiting types of arthritis, which tend to get better within two to three months,' says Isaacs. 'The problem is that with rheumatoid arthritis, two to three months is quite a long time, so by the time we know that the patients aren't going to get better, there can already be some significant damage to the joints.'

Making an early diagnosis of rheumatoid arthritis requires a battery of tests and a specialist doctor. But in most parts of the UK, patients must join the standard NHS waiting lists for these.

A group of specialists in Leeds, led by Professor Paul Emery, recognised this problem and were among the first people in the world to set up a rapid access clinic for suspected rheumatoid patients, which they called the Leeds Early Arthritis Project (LEAP). Emery and others went out into the community, made GPs aware of the initiative and educated them in spotting the early signs of the disease. The result is that patients are now seen in a fraction of the time that they would wait in other places. 'The early arthritis clinic is a fast-track system which depends on GP referrals,' says Isaacs. 'We would attempt to see people within two to three weeks.'

As well as seeing specialists, patients visiting the clinic have access to high-tech scanning equipment that can help in confirming a diagnosis. The first of these to be deployed in a clinical setting is musculoskeletal ultrasound – a modified form of the scans given to pregnant women. Although the technique is not unique to Leeds, Isaacs believes that the service there has been streamlined to provide better access. 'Leeds is different in that we train our rheumatologists to use ultrasound, and this helps us to fast-track because it means we don't depend on having a radiologist to do it for us.'

While people with suspected rheumatoid arthritis may not be able to go to rapid access clinics in other parts of the UK, their referrals should be prioritised. Most will be referred to the rheumatology department of the local hospital, and for a common disease like rheumatoid arthritis, Isaacs feels that a general rheumatologist is the best person to see. Of greater concern are the patients who are treated for some time by their GPs before being sent to a specialist.

'Although many GPs know a lot about rheumatoid, it is very much a developing area. If you look at practice today and practice ten years ago, it is completely different. So what we don't really like to see is a patient put on a simple anti-inflammatory drug for a few months before referral,' he says. 'That is what used to happen, but now if we see a patient in hospital and they are diagnosed with rheumatoid, they will immediately get put on a disease-modifying drug, which we use to try to slow the process down.'

Slowing the progression of rheumatoid arthritis in its early stages has become a priority, because if it is allowed to progress, the disease rapidly impacts on many areas of the patient's life. Among the most important of these is their ability to work. 'What people are becoming aware of is how many patients lose their jobs pretty early in the disease process; certainly within a year and often within six months,' says Isaacs.

Modern disease-modifying drugs are the treatments of choice for slowing rheumatoid arthritis, but this is a controversial area, as many of the latest and most effective treatments, such as anti-TNF drugs, are extremely expensive. Emery and his team are conducting research in this area, looking at whether using expensive drugs earlier can be cost-effective. 'Anti-TNF agents are very powerful new drugs, which at the moment we don't use immediately. One of the arguments for using them early might be if they do keep people in work, paying taxes and not having joint replacements. So we are looking at the impact of these therapies on work disability,' he says.

The benefits of rapid referral and diagnosis are apparent in this area as well, because under the current guidelines, anti-TNF drugs can only be given to patients who have tried and not responded to alternative treatments. By starting early and changing drugs quickly when they are ineffective, patients in Leeds can end up on the latest treatments early in the course of their disease. 'Patients in Leeds tend not just to get treated earlier, but when drugs are ineffective they get switched pretty rapidly. So we will have patients within a year of the onset of the disease who will be eligible for anti-TNF therapies,' says Isaacs.

While rapid access clinics have already become widespread for acute problems like cancer and stroke, they have been less readily adopted in the treatment of chronic illnesses. However, the success of the LEAP initiative in Leeds shows that they can also have a useful role to play in the treatment of rheumatoid arthritis.

Professor David Isenberg

For patients with severe or complex rheumatoid arthritis, or those with related but less well-known conditions such as lupus, Sjögren's syndrome and myositis, access to the very latest trials and treatments can be extremely beneficial. But this is only possible at a small number of centres in the UK. Professor David Isenberg is head of one of these: the University College Hospital Centre for Rheumatology. 'We are a secondary and tertiary referral centre,' he says, 'and we tend to deal with more complex cases and patients who have not been entirely satisfied with treatment elsewhere.'

Developing better treatments for diseases like rheumatoid arthritis involves a collaboration between scientists and doctors. Isenberg works at the interface between the two, bringing new treatments from the laboratory bench to the clinic. He has made a number of important contributions in this area.

In rheumatoid arthritis, for example, Isenberg and Professor Gabriel Panayi at Guy's Hospital were among the first in the world to begin treating patients with antibodies against tumour necrosis factor (TNF) alpha. TNF alpha plays an important part in causing inflammation and damage to joints in rheumatoid arthritis, and the antibodies act by blocking its effect. Patients given the new treatment experienced reduced inflammation and disability, together with a reduction in the rate of damage occurring to their joints.

More recently, Isenberg, in collaboration with Professor Jo Edwards, has been pioneering a new form of immunotherapy against lupus. In this technique, patients are injected with antibodies that specifically target the B-cells of the immune system, causing them to be destroyed. 'B-cells are at the centre of the mechanism by which lupus damages the body, so if you can stop the B-cells in their tracks, then this might stop the disease – at least temporarily,' he says.

In addition to benefiting from the latest research, the centre offers patients with less common disorders like lupus – which affects about one in every 3,500 people in the UK – a chance to see a real specialist in their condition. 'Colleagues at the district general hospitals may have a total of 30, 40 or 50 lupus patients, but they won't have the nearly 400 that I have seen,' he says.

Information collected from the large patient base flows back to inform the research at the centre. Isenberg recently reported a 20-year follow-up on 300 patients with lupus, some of whom have been under his care since the late 1970s. The follow-up study looked at the death rates for the patients and identified factors such as infection and vascular disease as major contributors to mortality. This type of information can be used to direct future scientific research towards the areas where it is most needed.

A long-term approach is also apparent in Isenberg's clinical work. 'I'm not very interested in seeing patients as a one-off and saying, "Well it's lupus, here's my advice for the next week or two, now go away,"' he says. Instead, the centre aims to provide a first-class clinical assessment followed by long-term care suited to the changing nature of the disease treated, which will often continue to affect patients for the rest of their lives. Some of those visiting the centre have 'shared care', which means that they are treated at their local hospitals as well as attending regular clinics in London.

In 1996, Isenberg was appointed as the Arthritis Research Campaign (ARC)'s Diamond Jubilee Professor of Rheumatology, reflecting a long-standing commitment to the organisation. 'I've served in a number of capacities over the last 15 years,' he says. 'I started off as a medical secretary for them back in 1987, and I've served on most of the ARC's committees. I am currently deputy chairman of the scientific coordinating committee, which is probably the most important, but I also serve on the academic development committee, which is peering into the future to see where academic thought might be needed.'

With this overview of the field, Isenberg has a positive message for sufferers of these debilitating diseases. 'There are a huge number of advances going on in most of the major autoimmune diseases, particularly rheumatoid arthritis and lupus,' he says, 'and I have no doubt that in five or ten years' time we will be doing things rather differently from the way we are at the moment.'

Dr Tim Spector

In his research, Dr Tim Spector, a consultant rheumatologist at St Thomas' Hospital in London is looking at the causes of osteoporosis, osteoarthritis and other rheumatic diseases. He is based at the St Thomas' Hospital Twin Research Unit, where he studies the development of these diseases in identical and non-identical twins to ascertain the extent of their genetic component.

'We are looking at the similarity in the identicals compared to the similarity in the non-identicals. Both groups are brought up together and have similar sharing of environments, but the identical twins share all their genes, non-identicals only half. The difference can only be due to a genetic effect. Our first discovery was that osteoarthritis, which was thought to be due mainly to being overweight, playing too much sport or the general wear and tear of ageing, is actually around 60 per cent genetic.'

The St Thomas' group are now trying to determine which genes predispose a person to one of these rheumatic diseases. Once this is known, it could be used to assess more accurately who is at risk and to develop better treatments.

Linked to his research is Spector's concern that the elderly, who are at greatest risk from osteoporosis, are not getting access to treatment on the NHS because of a chronic shortage of bone density scanners and a traditional approach among some doctors that focuses predominantly on women around the menopause.

'The over-60s group, who are at high risk of fractures – particularly people with previous fractures or with family histories – are not being picked up and sent for screening,' says Spector. 'When around 70,000 people have a wrist fracture every year, and less than 5 per cent get referred to osteoporosis clinics despite a threefold increased risk of further fractures, you know something is going wrong.'

Osteoporosis is often thought of in association with the menopause, and many women are referred for scans around this time, despite the fact that their overall risk of developing osteoporosis is extremely low. This would not be a problem, except that the scanners used to detect bone density, which are called dual energy X-ray absorptiometry (DXA) scanners, are in extremely short supply, and consequently waiting times are long. 'We have got the lowest number of DXA scanners in Europe, and a lot of them are paid for by research or drug companies rather than the Trusts themselves,' he says. 'Some patients have a 12-month wait.'

'Some cases of osteoporosis are barn door. For example, if you are having multiple fractures, you don't need a bone density scan before you go on treatment. But other cases are more complicated, and it is bad practice to start treating people with drugs without being sure of a diagnosis, which happens in some places.'

Elderly patients who show up at casualty with fractures are often not referred to specialist osteoporosis clinics because systems for picking up these warning signs are not in place. Spector thinks that this is an area where patients can take steps to improve their own care. 'In many instances, it is not clear whose responsibility it is to make the referral. Is it the hospital casualty department's job? Is it the GP's job? The system is falling short, so this is an area where patients themselves, or their relatives, can be proactive and ask their GPs for a referral.'

The referral ideally should be to a specialist osteoporosis clinic or at least a rheumatologist with an interest in the condition, as there is no guarantee that a general rheumatologist will have experience in treating the disease. 'Ten years ago, rheumatologists did not treat osteoporosis; it was left to endocrinologists and gynaecologists,' says Spector. 'So it has only been in the last ten years that it has come into the training for most places. You still find old rheumatologists who are seeing people with a condition they haven't ever been trained in.'

Establishing whether someone has a special interest in osteoporosis can be difficult, but leading charities in the area, such as the National Osteoporosis Society, can provide useful information for patients. 'They know where most of the scanners are and would be able to tell you if the lead clinician has a particular interest in osteoporosis or not. If your hospital is on the list, you are fine, but if it is not, you don't necessarily know whether they are good or bad, so you might have to do your own research,' he says.

The internet is useful for patients trying to find out about their doctors, as sites like Pub Med (www.ncbi.nlm.nih.gov/entrez) can reveal an individual's areas of research. Being active in research is a good indicator that a doctor has current knowledge of the field. 'If they have written anything, even if it is a little review or something, it shows they must be keeping themselves up to date because they would be going to all the meetings. If they are on advisory boards or have connections with the industry, that is another sign they know what is going on. There are some good clinicians who don't publish, but who are conscientious about going to meetings. Usually they will have some affiliation with an organisation such as the Arthritis and Rheumatism Council or the National Osteoporosis Society.'

Although research initiatives like the one at St Thomas' are likely to lead to better treatments for osteoporosis, they can only produce maximum benefit if they are targeted correctly. That means improving systems for picking up risk groups like the elderly and better provision of diagnostic facilities.

Professor Pat Woo

The outlook for children with rheumatic diseases has improved a great deal in the last 10 or 20 years, partly because of work done by Professor Pat Woo and her team at the Centre for Paediatric and Adolescent Rheumatology at the Great Ormond Street and Middlesex hospitals in London. However, Woo feels that access to specialist paediatric rheumatologists is inconsistent across the country, and some children with chronic arthritis are treated at their local hospitals for too long before getting to a specialist centre.

'There are black spots and there are good places,' she says. 'The south-east is not brilliant because Great Ormond Street is the only big unit, though we are trying to set up satellites now. Certainly, doctors know of our unit at Great Ormond Street, but patients might stay longer in secondary care here than in other places.'

Rheumatic diseases are not often thought of as a cause of illness in children, but they are more common than most people believe. Around 1 in 1,000 children suffers from arthritis that stays for more than six weeks in the same joint, and while the other diseases in the group are rarer, they can be significantly debilitating or even fatal in some cases.

Despite their severity, treatments are improving. For example, Woo's department at Great Ormond Street, which is the largest of its type in the world, has been active in research into juvenile arthritis and juvenile dermatomyositis – a chronic and progressive disease that causes skin rashes, lesions, muscle weakness and other problems in children as young as eight or nine – and the death rate is now falling. 'If you look at the old books, the mortality rate for dermatomyositis is 30 per cent, but it doesn't need to be that high if treated properly, and we certainly don't have that figure. We run a big research programme to try to find the causes of the disease, and we have also set up a network of UK and European centres so that we can do clinical trials,' she says.

By far the most common type of juvenile arthritis is the acute form of the disease. This often occurs as the result of infection, and it can be successfully treated by a good general paediatrician without referral to a tertiary centre. 'There are acute arthritic diseases that kids get after an obvious viral infection or bug, and they usually get better within six weeks,' says Woo. 'But the cases that don't have an infectious trigger are the ones that can go on for a long time, and it is then that patients should be put in touch with tertiary centres or paediatric rheumatologists.'

The main area where a specialist can offer a better service for children with juvenile idiopathic arthritis (the long-lasting form of the disease) is in drug and rehabilitation therapies. Treatments such as steroids are well known, but their effects – and side-effects – are highly dependent on how they are used. 'Drug therapy is crucial and how you use your drugs is very important,' she says. 'How you use steroids makes all the difference sometimes, and the specialist will know more about that than the general paediatrician.'

In the past, finding an appropriate specialist in this situation could be problematic. But in 1994, after pressure from Woo and others, the Royal College of Physicians and the Royal College of Paediatrics and Child Health recognised paediatric rheumatology as a specialty in its own right, separate from orthopaedics, paediatrics and rheumatology. The colleges now have a specialist register of consultants who have trained in the area, which parents or doctors can refer to if they wish to ensure that the person they are seeing is an expert. 'It is getting much better than it was. Fifteen years ago, paediatric rheumatology wasn't even a recognised specialty, whereas now it has its own training and specialist requirements,' says Woo.

Another potential source of information for parents is the Children with Chronic Arthritis Association (CCAA), which is a national support network. As well as advising on where the various centres of expertise are, the CCAA can help with the more day-to-day problems faced by parents. 'I think a lot of parents find it very useful because they can talk to other parents about their problems, including simple questions like, "My child won't take this colour medicine, what do I do?"' she says.

The CCAA and the Arthritis Research Campaign are also useful for parents who want to find out about their child's condition before seeing a specialist, as the literature they produce tends to be more accurate than other sources, such as the internet.

There have been improvements in both the treatments and the organisation of services for sufferers of childhood rheumatic diseases, but their causes remain poorly understood. In around two-thirds of cases of juvenile chronic arthritis, the disease will go into remission with the aid of appropriate therapy by the time they reach adulthood. In order to get the best out of the drug therapies available, it is important that children with these diseases get to see a paediatric rheumatologist at a specialist centre.

Asthma

What is the specialty?

Respiratory medicine, or for children, respiratory paediatrics or, more rarely, clinical allergy.

What is asthma and how many people does it affect?

Asthma is a condition affecting the bronchi, small tubes that carry air in and out of the lungs. Most people with asthma are atopic; that is, they have a tendency to allergy (although there is a lack of consensus among doctors as to how important a role allergy plays in asthma; see Kay, p.74–5; Thomson, p.76–8; Warner, p.79–81). Exposure to certain stimuli such as cold air, respiratory infections, smoke and environmental pollutants, sudden changes in temperature and vigorous exercise can trigger an asthma attack, during which the lining of the bronchi becomes inflamed and swollen. This in turn causes a restriction of airflow and leads to wheezing, coughing and tightness in the chest. Attacks can last from minutes to days, and in severe cases may be life-threatening.

The incidence of asthma is on the rise all over the world. Around 10 per cent of people have had an attack of asthma at some time in their lives, and in the UK an estimated 8 million people have been diagnosed with the condition. Of these, some 5.1 million people (one in eight children and one in thirteen adults) in the UK are currently being treated. For reasons that doctors still don't understand, some people (possibly around 5 per cent) have a type of asthma that can't be well controlled even when they take maximum doses of asthma medication.

Some 1,500 people die from asthma each year, over one-third of whom are under 65. Asthma is the most common long-term childhood illness, with one in five children having been diagnosed with asthma at some time during childhood, and one in eight receiving treatment. Despite its prevalence, parents of children with asthma do not always get the professional support and help they need.

How is it currently treated?

The aims of asthma treatment are to control the symptoms of asthma attacks when they happen, to improve lung function and to prevent the condition from worsening, using the minimum medication with the fewest side-effects, and to provide the information people need to enable them to manage their own condition (self-management).

Control and management

Assessing the control and management of asthma may involve the following:

- **Monitoring your peak expiratory flow (PEF):** done by blowing a special meter that indicates how open the airways are. The more expanded the airways are, the higher the rate at which air can be expired from the lungs and the higher the peak flow reading.

- **Reversibility test:** your peak flow reading will be taken followed by a dose of reliever medication. After 25 minutes your peak flow will be recorded again. The results will give some indication as to how well the reliever opens up your airways.

- **Spirometry:** a piece of equipment called a spirometer can be used to measure your lung function.

- **Trial of treatment:** this may include a two-week course of steroid tablets to see if your lung function improves by reducing inflammation (see also Chung, p.69).

Medications

The current mainstays of asthma treatment are inhaled medications designed to bring symptoms under control when an attack happens, and other inhaled drugs designed to control and help reduce the frequency of attacks.

- **Reliever inhalation (bronchodilators).** These drugs include salbutamol and terbutaline sulphate. An active asthma attack is treated with inhaled drugs known as bronchodilators, which relax muscle and open the airways, making it easier to breathe again. Most relievers are fast-acting, usually taking five to ten minutes to bring relief. However some, for example salmeterol and eformoterol, are long-acting, with effects lasting up to 12 hours. Everyone with asthma should carry a reliever inhaler (usually blue in colour) to take in the event of an acute attack.

- **Preventive inhalation.** Although many people with mild, occasional asthma may manage with reliever inhalation as their only treatment, if you have continuous or severe symptoms, you will also need to take regular preventer inhalation to control swelling and inflammation of the airways and to desensitise the airways to asthma triggers. Taking preventer treatment regularly improves the long-term control of asthma and reduces the risk of permanently damaging the airways. Most preventer inhalers are brown, red or orange. Inhaled steroids – for example, beclomethasone dipropionate, fluticasone propionate and budesonide – are long-acting anti-inflammatory drugs that help reduce the inflammation that causes asthma. Effects last for around 12 hours, so they are taken twice a day.

There is a wide choice of different inhalers on the market, the most common one being the aerosol or metered dose inhaler commonly known as a 'puffer'. There are also a number of dry powder inhalers and breath-activated inhalers, which people sometimes prefer because they do not require the coordination needed to use a puffer. People who need higher dosages of inhaled steroids can develop a sore mouth or hoarseness, and for this reason may be recommended to use an aerosol inhaler with a plastic 'spacer' device, which ensures that the drug ends up in the lungs rather than the mouth and reduces the risks of these side-effects. Spacers are also used for young children for both reliever and preventive inhalation.

- **Severe asthma.** If your asthma is severe, you may be referred to a specialist who can prescribe other, stronger treatments. These may include oral or inhaled steroids in a preventative role and immunosuppressive drugs (drugs that suppress the immune system) such as cyclosporin, methotrexate and immunoglobulin. If you are prescribed these, you will need to be monitored closely by a respiratory specialist.

How does this measure up to treatment in the rest of the world?

Guidelines for the management of asthma in adults and children drawn up by the British Thoracic Society have been in existence for the past 12 years. The latest ones are in the pipeline and should be available in late 2002 (see Doull, p.73). The guidelines recommend a stepwise approach, by which medications are added on an 'as and when needed' basis to achieve the best possible control. The basic guidelines are remarkably similar to those in western Europe, Australia, New Zealand and the USA. However, asthma is classified differently in the USA, and inhaled steroids are not so popular as they are in the UK. So, whereas in the UK chronic asthma is graded according to the amount of medication needed to keep symptoms under control, in the USA asthma is classified by its severity. People with asthma in the USA are more likely to see an allergist or clinical immunologist than in the UK, which only has around 90 NHS allergy clinics (see Warner, p.79).

What new treatments are available?

Two fairly new inhaled corticosteroids have been introduced:

- **Qvar Inhalation Aerosol.** A CFC-free aerosol containing beclomethasone diproprionate.
- **Advair Discus (seretide).** Another preventer, which comes in the form of a combination powder medicine that combines an inhaled corticosteroid (fluticasone propionate) with an inhaled long-acting drug that dilates the bronchi (salameterol).

Also fairly new are long-acting bronchodilator treatments such as formoterol, a type of beta-blocker (drugs which affect nerve transmissions), the effects of which last for around 12 hours.

There is also a new class of preventers known as leukotriene modifiers, which come in the form of a tablet that is taken once or twice a day. The tablets block the effect of chemicals called leukotrienes, which are released from the lung cells of people with asthma and play a part in inflammation. The first of these, montelukast, was launched in the UK in 1998.

Can I get these on the NHS?

Several CFC-free reliever inhalers are available and others are being phased in gradually. One CFC-free preventer inhaler is also available. There are currently two leukotriene modifiers on the market in the UK. The first, montelukast (Singulair), which is taken once daily, is prescribed for adults and children aged over two. You can get it on the NHS, but only as an adjunct to inhalation treatment for people whose asthma is not well controlled using low-dose inhaled steroids, to enable the dose of steroid to be reduced. The second, zafirlukast (Accolate), is taken twice daily, and is currently prescribed only for patients aged over 12. Like montelukast, it is usually given as an adjunct to preventers, although it may be prescribed as an alternative to inhaled preventers for some people with mild asthma, for whom inhaled steroids aren't suitable.

What treatments are in the pipeline?

The main classes of drugs for treating asthma have been used for over 20 years now. However, we could be on the brink of a revolution in asthma treatment with the discoveries of genetic research. Many doctors think this could lead to major advances in the understanding of the underlying origins of asthma and to new treatments in the next few years. A number of drugs are already in the final stages of development. These include other leuokotriene modifiers (see p.60), and other drugs aimed at blocking substances involved in the inflammatory reaction.

Also in development is a new class of asthma medications called anti-IgE, which block the production of immunoglobulin E, a molecule produced by the body that recognises specific allergens (substances you are allergic to). IgE resides in the nose, lungs and skin, and when you are exposed to something you are allergic to, the allergen binds to IgE and sparks off an allergic reaction. The first anti-IgE medication, omalizumab, is given in injection form every two weeks and is undergoing clinical trials. It's thought it may be particularly useful for long-term treatment of people with moderate to severe allergic asthma and could reduce the frequency of attacks, lower the doses of steroids needed and improve quality of life.

Scientists are also researching new, less risky 'desensitisation' therapies. Desensitisation involves identifying substances that spark attacks (allergens) and then giving a series of injections over a period of weeks designed to enable the body to build up resistence to that allergen – in effect, vaccinating against asthma. The treatment was formerly used most often for people with troublesome hay fever, but has largely been abandoned in recent years because of its potential to cause life-threatening reactions. For the past few years it has been used only in specialist centres for people with extreme allergic reactions (anaphylaxis) to, say, bee stings. However, doctors are now revisiting the treatment, and researchers are looking to refine the process within the next three to five years (see Kay, p.74–5).

There is also collaboration underway between doctors, architects and environmental engineers to investigate whether novel ventilation systems can reduce the level of house dust mites in homes. It is hoped that this avenue will produce a clinical improvement for patients without the need for drug therapy (see Thomson, p.78).

Who treats it?

Diagnosis and treatment will usually be under the supervision of your GP. A number of GPs have a special interest in asthma and some run dedicated asthma clinics with specialist asthma nurses, who have further training in asthma care (see Doull, p.72–3). If you are one of the 5 per cent of asthma sufferers whose condition cannot be controlled by using medication, your GP should refer you to a consultant in respiratory medicine or an allergy specialist.

What training will the specialist have?

Before becoming a consultant, your doctor will have had a general medical training, which includes five years at university followed by one year as a House Officer, before gaining registration with the General Medical Council. They will then have spent two to three years as a Senior House Officer in various medical disciplines. This is followed by a five- or six-year period of specialist registrar training, working in different hospitals, leading to a Certificate of Completion of Specialist Training that is recognised throughout Europe. In the fifth year and post-certification, doctors are encouraged to train to become sub-specialists.

For a respiratory specialist, their registrar training will have been in respiratory medicine. For a clinical immunologist or allergy specialist, it will have been in immunology.

Where will I receive care?

At the GP's surgery, asthma clinic or, for severe, uncontrolled asthma, at a respiratory clinic or specialist NHS allergy clinic. Children with severe, uncontrolled asthma may need to be admitted to hospital. This will normally be done via your GP, although in the case of a severe acute attack it will probably be safer to go straight to the hospital. If your child has severe asthma or has had to be admitted to hospital several times previously, you may be able to agree with the specialist that your child can go straight to the respiratory or paediatric ward without going via your GP.

What questions should I ask about my treatment?

- How often should I come to the asthma clinic?
- What will happen at the asthma clinic?
- What reliever treatment will be prescribed and when should I (my child) use it?
- Is it short-acting or long-acting?
- What preventer treatment are you prescribing and when should I (my child) use it?
- Are inhaled steroids safe?
- Will I (my child) experience side-effects and what might these be?
- What kind of inhaler will I (my child) be using and how should I (my child) use it?
- Are there any oral treatments you can prescribe?
- Should I (my child) have an allergy test?
- What about desensitisation treatment?
- How will I know if my (my child's) asthma is getting worse?
- What should I do if my (my child's) asthma gets worse?
- How do I know if it is an emergency?
- Should I go to the hospital if I (my child) has an asthma attack?
- How will I know when I (my child) am better?
- What can I do to make sure I (my child) stays better?
- How will asthma affect what I (my child) can do?
- How can I (my child) avoid triggers that make the asthma worse?
- Can I (my child) exercise with asthma?
- Can I (my child) go camping/go on holiday?
- Will asthma affect my job?
- Can I take my asthma medications if I am pregnant/breastfeeding?

What will my treatment involve?

Treatment involves avoiding anything that triggers your asthma and taking your reliever and preventer medicines, plus self-monitoring with a peak flow meter. You or your child should be seen periodically at a dedicated asthma clinic, usually at the GP's surgery and more rarely at the hospital, to check on your medication, your inhaler technique and to monitor for any side-effects. Exactly how often you attend the clinic will depend on the nature of your asthma and how severe it is. If you experience asthma only at certain times, for example during the hayfever season, you may need to have an appointment only once a year. If, on the other hand, your asthma is severe and difficult to control, you will probably need to attend the clinic every month or couple of months.

Every GP should keep an asthma register; a document, or more usually today a computerised file, that includes details of your asthma and how it is being managed.

If you (or your child) have a severe acute asthma attack that you are unable to bring under control, you will need to be admitted to hospital, where you will be given oxygen and a high dose of steroids by mouth to control symptoms. In extreme cases you may need to be admitted to intensive care. Once your asthma has been brought under control, the specialist will try to identify why your asthma has become worse; for example, whether it is a result of poor technique in using your inhaler or of not following your personal asthma management plan. Before discharging you they may adjust your reliever treatment and increase your preventer treatment if necessary, as well as weaning you off any oral steroids that may have been prescribed. Once you go home the specialist should let your GP have details of your attack, and the GP should contact you within a week. The specialist should also make arrangements for you to have a follow-up appointment in two to four weeks.

What makes a REAL difference to getting better?
There is currently no cure for asthma, although some children do grow out of it. The key to successful control lies in learning how and when to adjust your treatment in response to changes in the condition.
- **Having a GP with a real interest in asthma.** Your GP has a key role to play in diagnosing your condition and in starting you on the right treatment. Ideally, they should run a dedicated asthma clinic where you (or your child) can go for regular checks and have your treatment monitored. If your GP doesn't appear to be interested in asthma, you should ask to be referred to a respiratory or allergy specialist at the hospital.

- **Having a personal asthma plan.** A huge number of studies over the past two decades have proved that having a written personal asthma plan reduces symptoms, improves lung function, reduces the frequency of attacks, reduces the need for reliever treatment and oral steroids, reduces the inappropriate use of antibiotics and improves the quality of life. The plan should outline how and when to use your medication, what to do if asthma symptoms get worse and what steps you should take before seeking medical help. The National Asthma Campaign (see p.68) produces a pack called *Be in Control*, which includes a personalised asthma plan.
- **Lifestyle modification.** Stopping smoking and learning to avoid or limit exposure to triggers such as colds and viral infections, pets, tobacco smoke, house dust mites and pollen are important parts of taking control of asthma. Keeping a personal trigger diary in which you note down what seems to bring on symptoms or exacerbate asthma is extremely valuable. You should show this to the GP or asthma nurse. Exercise can worsen asthma. However, that doesn't mean you shouldn't exercise. Your GP can advise you on how to prevent asthma symptoms from interfering with exercise.
- **Teamwork.** A good working partnership between you, your GP, asthma nurse and specialist is the basis of effective asthma treatment. In the case of a child, the health visitor and/or school nurse will also need to be involved. Your child's school should also have a proper written asthma policy in place.

What is the difference between a well-run and a badly run asthma clinic?

Clinics vary slightly from one GP's practice to the next and from hospital to hospital. According to the British Thoracic Society, the aims of a good asthma service are to prevent asthma attacks, to reduce the amount of illness caused by asthma and reduce the number of deaths caused by asthma. A well-run clinic should include:

Expert staff

This should include a GP with special knowledge of and interest in asthma, or a specialist plus one or more specialist nurses who have had extra training in the management of asthma.

Practical information

The clinic should provide you with practical information on all aspects of asthma, including the use of your inhaler, how to perform peak flow readings and how to recognise if your (or your child's) asthma is worsening, as well as what to do in an emergency.

Time to talk

Clinic appointments should be long enough for you to discuss your (or your child's) asthma and how it affects your life, and to raise any worries or concerns you may have about the condition or its treatment.

Personal management plan

You should always be given a written personal management plan (see p.65).

Regular follow-up

The clinic should have a well-organised system that enables you to have your symptoms reviewed at regular intervals to make sure that your asthma is under control and that the medication you are receiving remains appropriate.

Will I get better treatment if I go privately?

Not in terms of pharmacological treatments, which will be identical to those prescribed on the NHS. Where you may do better if you decide to consult a specialist privately is that you will be able to see the same doctor every time you make an appointment and build up a relationship with him or her. You're also likely to get more frequent review appointments – say, every six months – as well as having more time at each appointment to explore factors that may affect your tendency to have asthma attacks, such as pets, stress or environmental factors. Acute asthma attacks are most usually managed within the NHS, as most private hospitals are not set up for dealing with emergencies.

Will I get better treatment if I go abroad?

Asthma guidelines are fairly similar in Europe and the USA, so you are unlikely to get very different treatment if you go abroad. What's more, because of the nature of asthma and the potential need for emergency treatment, it's usually better to be treated locally.

What support will I be offered by the clinic and are there any independent support groups I can join?

The clinic should offer you regular follow-up appointments and provide written information leaflets about various aspects of asthma. They should be able to put you in touch with any local self-help groups.

Useful addresses

For information on NHS and private allergy clinics contact:

Allergy UK (formerly The British Allergy Foundation)
Deepdene House
30 Bellegrove Road
Welling
Kent DA16 3PY
Tel 020 8303 8525
Helpline 020 8303 8583 (9 am to 9 pm Monday to Friday,
10 am to 1 pm Saturday and Sunday)
www.allergyuk.org

British Lung Foundation
78 Hatton Garden
London EC1N 8LD
Tel 020 7831 5831
www.lunguk.org

British Thoracic Society
17 Doughty Street
London WC1N 2PL
Tel 020 7831 8778
www.brit-thoracic.org.uk

National Asthma Campaign
Providence House
Providence Place
London N1 0NT
Tel 020 7226 2260
Helpline 0845 701 0203 (9 am to 7 pm Monday to Friday)
www.asthmaplus.org.uk

Expert opinions

Professor K F Chung

Understanding the precise details of your asthma and what is likely to provoke an attack are important steps towards successful management of the disease. Kian Fan Chung, a consultant respiratory physician at the Royal Brompton Hospital in London and Professor of Respiratory Medicine at the National Heart and Lung Institute, Imperial College, co-chairs the PARA UK group, which is investigating the factors that can induce asthma attacks.

For patients with severe asthma, having a serious attack is a constant source of worry, especially for those with 'brittle asthma', whose condition can deteriorate in as little as five minutes.

In 2001, the PARA UK group published results of a study on 163 at-risk, severe asthma patients, which revealed respiratory infections, exercise and cold air to be the commonest triggers of asthma attacks. Laughter, taking aspirin and allergies were also reported as triggers, and one in ten female sufferers said that their asthma episodes were related to their menstrual cycles.

The group is now attempting to better understand these triggers and to find new ones by recruiting a much larger number of patients. 'We hope to collect about 2,000 patients and see if we can pick up any patterns,' says Chung. 'The point of doing all this is so that in the future we will be able to tell patients what is provoking the attacks and advise them on avoidance measures.'

Better control of asthma can also be achieved by understanding the day-to-day variations in its activity. Chung and his team are developing tests for asthma and other respiratory conditions that may provide doctors with a fast and accurate way of establishing how active the disease is in each patient.

'We are developing non-invasive tests,' says Chung. 'Tests that take bits of tissue from the lungs are invasive; you have to put a tube inside the lungs. Non-invasive tests are easy to do and more acceptable to the patient. For example, you can ask a patient to blow into a machine and sample for nitric oxide, which is a gas, in the air they blow out. Nitric oxide is valuable because its levels are increased in patients with asthma, and we're hoping we can use it as a marker to tell us how active the asthma is. If the level is high, we may have to give more treatment. This sort of measurement may prove to be better than asking the patient, "How are you feeling today?"'

In addition to asthma patients, Chung sees people with persistent respiratory symptoms such as cough, shortness of breath and wheezing, with conditions ranging from bronchitis to chronic obstructive airways disease. These conditions all involve inflammation of the airways, and his research focuses on understanding how this occurs. 'In most respiratory conditions, you have some form of inflammation in the lungs,' he says. 'I'm interested in how the inflammation translates into damage and symptoms. Basically, you have to understand how the inflammation occurs and what is happening so you can try to control it. You need to know what's happening before you can intervene.'

Because every patient's asthma is different, there are numerous forms of treatment available both to relieve symptoms and to prevent attacks from occurring. Given this complexity, Chung feels that patients with some understanding of their condition can get more out of their consultations with a hospital specialist. 'Patients need to learn about the condition they have. The sort of things that are important to ask are, "What treatments are there? What are the side-effects of treatment? What do you expect to get from the treatment? When is it going to work? How long am I going to be on it? And what is the prognosis for the next ten years?"' he says.

It can be worthwhile to ask about the unit as well, as there are a number of areas where a specialist centre, like the Royal Brompton, can offer additional services. 'We have access to new treatments,' he says. 'We also have facilities for research, special tests – for example, bronchoscopies or methods for measuring inflammation – and for observation.'

'Another thing is that we have a bit more time to devote to patients with severe problems, and because we don't have the same time pressure we are more thorough. We leave no stone unturned. People in general hospitals are often just too busy to have special interests. In many instances, when a patient comes to see you, they haven't had someone sit them down, go through the facts and calm their worries. If you're a general physician and not an expert in the area, you won't be able to provide them with this.'

As an expert in the condition, Chung feels that there are genuine reasons for optimism. Despite the fact that asthma affects people for many years, and curative treatments are still some way off, patients can look forward to improved testing that allows therapies to be more closely targeted to disease activity and a better understanding of what triggers asthma attacks.

Dr Iolo Doull

Many children with asthma do not take their medicines as instructed, increasing the risk of hospitalisation or even, in extreme cases, death. Despite efforts to improve patient education, the problem has doctors stumped, says Dr Iolo Doull, a consultant in paediatric respiratory medicine at the University Hospital of Wales. 'Knowing more about asthma does not mean that you are more likely to take your medicine,' he says. 'It is something that we all worry about now: increasing education does not seem to make any difference.'

Studies in children using puffers fitted with a chip that records when the medicine was taken have produced some startling results. 'If you see 100 patients with asthma,' says Doull, '33 will take their medicine regularly on time, 33 will take it very irregularly, just here and there, and 33 won't take it at all. So no matter how good our medicines are, if the patient won't take it, we are not going to win. Only about half of all children take their medicine as directed, while the others take it very infrequently, and sometimes not at all.'

Medicines used to treat asthma fall into two broad categories: relievers and preventers. Relievers, such as steroids, act rapidly to reduce the symptoms of asthma, while preventers are used to control the disease in the longer term. Because preventers do not have an immediately apparent effect, children with asthma are particularly unlikely to use them as directed. But that can expose them to substantial risks. 'In mild asthma, death is mercifully very uncommon, but hospitalisations are more frequent. Severe asthmatics may actually be putting themselves – their lives – at risk.'

The focus of asthma care is shifting to address this problem. One initiative has been the widespread introduction of clinics run by specialist asthma nurses in GP surgeries, and Doull feels that these nurse-led clinics can be more effective than seeing a specialist in getting a child's asthma under control. 'The vast majority of children with asthma do not need to come close to hospital, and it would be wrong if they did,' he says. 'Many children don't need to see their GP regularly, as most asthma is managed very well by asthma nurses. If you look at hospital admissions for asthma in the last five or ten years, they are decreasing across the UK, and I suspect that one of the major factors in this is the move towards nurse-led asthma management.'

Doull feels that this improvement can be attributed partly to the establishment of a set of guidelines for asthma care laid down by the British Thoracic Society. 'If you are looking at a system with clear guidelines,' he says, 'nurses will go with those guidelines much better than doctors, who always like to try to do their own thing. Nurses are also able to monitor patients better and get a closer feel for each individual because they see their patients more regularly.'

In some severe asthma cases, or where the disease is not being controlled effectively in primary care, it can become necessary to see a specialist, usually a general paediatrician for a child's asthma. Doull's advice to patients in this situation is to ensure that they are seeing the paediatric department's lead doctor for respiratory conditions. 'The other thing to stress is that most GPs see more asthma than do general paediatricians. GPs see it regularly, while the number of asthmatics going to hospital may be relatively small. So, if you are being referred, you definitely want to see someone who has an interest in respiratory diseases.'

Whatever the level of expertise of the specialist, however, treatments for asthma are only going to be effective if they are taken appropriately. And with patient education appearing to have limited benefit, researchers are looking at other ways to improve compliance. 'There is going to be a move towards combination therapy,' says Doull. 'Combinations of inhaled steroids and long-term preventers will become much more widespread in the next few years. With combinations, because they are both a reliever and a preventer, people tend to use them when they feel unwell. And when they take them, they are not only relieving their symptoms, they are also preventing further attacks.'

Professor A Barry Kay

Professor Barry Kay and his colleagues at the National Heart and Lung Institute in London are refining a 100-year-old form of treatment that is still almost unique in offering the potential for a long-lasting cure for people suffering from allergic conditions such as allergic asthma or hay fever. He feels that the technique, which is called immunotherapy, has been neglected in the UK relative to other countries.

'Hay fever responds very well to immunotherapy, but there is nowhere in this country, with one or two exceptions, where you can get this form of treatment; whereas if you go to continental Europe, the United States or Japan, it is fairly freely available. It is just amazing, the negative attitude to allergy amongst the medical establishment in this country.'

The technique of immunotherapy is fairly straightforward. Usually, a crude extract of the substance that triggers the allergy or allergen is given to patients by injection in increasing doses. Generally, this is effective in reducing the allergy, but it can trigger a severe, even occasionally fatal, allergic reaction called an anaphylaxis, which is why it has fallen out of general use.

Kay's interest in the area has been in identifying the small sections of the allergen that are responsible for reducing the allergy. These fragments, or peptides, can then be used in immunotherapy, reducing the risk of anaphylaxis. 'It is thought that if you inject an allergen in the form of a small peptide rather than the whole molecule, the immune system recognises that it is different from the whole allergen,' he says.

Once inside the body, the peptides appear to act on the T-cells of the immune system, which have a central role in generating the allergic response. 'The T-cell, instead of expanding and doing nasty things, just curls up – it doesn't actually die but it goes into non-cooperative mode,' says Kay. 'The treatment also seems to recruit a different type of T-cell, called a T-regulatory cell, which dampens down the allergic response.'

Different people respond to different peptides due to variations in their genes. So Kay and his colleagues, in collaboration with a large vaccine company, have developed a vaccine that contains a selection of these peptides, covering most of the population. Early results are promising, but Kay points out that they are still some way from a safe and effective treatment. 'We have got a lot of things to iron out,' he says. 'For example, we want to make sure it is long-lasting and we want to get the dose right.'

Kay believes that the widespread neglect of allergy extends to all levels of care. 'Asthma is like other chronic diseases, in that generally it is difficult to get an expert opinion quickly. You can go to your GP, and GPs are in a strong position because they have got some very effective treatments such as inhaled corticosteroids and bronchodilators,' he says. 'What the GPs don't have is the access to allergy services, which would help them to find specific allergies and advise on allergy avoidance. This is something of a defect in our system at present.'

Another problem is that there is a lack of consensus among doctors as to how important a role allergy plays in conditions like asthma. But Kay feels that attitudes are changing. 'It depends on who you talk to,' he says. 'If you talk to established chest physicians, who see lots of patients with chronic asthma, they say allergy is not important. But if you talk to younger people who are interested in the field, it is clear that allergy is significant, and allergy-avoidance measures, such as reducing house dust mite levels and identifying triggers like pets or pollen, can be helpful.'

While the medical profession is beginning to recognise a need for more comprehensive allergy services, Kay feels that competition for funding from other, higher-profile areas such as cancer make it likely that any changes will be gradual. This could lead to UK patients missing out on advances in allergy treatments, such as the safer immunotherapy techniques being pioneered at the Royal Brompton.

Professor Neil Thomson

A good hospital asthma service depends at least as much on its supporting staff and facilities as it does on its consultants, says Neil Thomson, who is Professor of Respiratory Medicine at the University of Glasgow and a respiratory consultant at Gartnavel General Hospital. 'I think it is fair to say that most general respiratory physicians would have a wide experience of dealing with asthma,' he says. 'But I think it is important to find out what additional support there is.'

The investigations and tests used to diagnose asthma are not particularly high-tech, and should be readily available at most units. However, having specialist nurses, established links to physiotherapy and a well-defined system for patient education and support can be instrumental in achieving good asthma control. 'The expertise of paramedical staff, and a focus on patient expectations and inhaler technique are all very important aspects of assessing patients with asthma. It is also useful to find out what support they have from the physiotherapy department, as some patients with asthma can over-breathe, and, for them, seeing a physiotherapist can be helpful.'

One area where consultant expertise can make a difference is in allergy, which is often an important trigger of asthma attacks. 'It is a factor that patients are often interested in,' says Thomson, 'and I think I would want to know what experience or interest my consultant has in the allergic aspects of asthma.'

Only a small proportion of asthma sufferers need to be seen by a hospital specialist at all, as most mild to moderate cases can be managed effectively in the community. But there are several groups who should ask for a referral. 'About 20 per cent of patients have more severe asthma, which is much harder to control, and they would benefit from seeing a specialist. Then there are patients in whom it is not clear whether it is asthma or not, as there are other common causes of breathlessness such as heart disease and chronic obstructive pulmonary disease. A specialist can make a diagnosis before passing the patient back to the GP for further management. There is a group, too, who have occupational symptoms. For example, bakers can become sensitised to flour. They are quite difficult to assess and are probably better seen by a specialist.'

For people who are seeing a specialist, Thomson thinks that some simple preparation can make the consultation much more productive. 'If they are concerned about trigger factors, such as allergies or stress, it is often helpful for the patient to list those before seeing their specialist. It is also useful to consider what day-to-day activities they have problems with, because, again, the doctor who is seeing them can give information about that. Patients are also often interested in complementary medicines, so it is important to raise that with the consultant. It is also helpful to the specialist if patients bring the inhaler they are using with them to the clinic, as well as a list of all drug medications.'

Thomson's holistic approach to asthma treatment is reflected in a wide range of research interests. In the laboratory, he is trying to find out why steroid drugs, which are widely used to treat asthma, are less effective in asthma sufferers who smoke. 'We have found that individuals who are cigarette smokers don't respond as well to inhaled steroids, and we are looking at the mechanisms of that. Obviously, we advise asthmatics who smoke to give up, but in those who have difficulty, this research has implications as to whether they should consider other forms of treatment.'

The group has also shown that asthma patients taking high doses of inhaled steroids over long periods of time can have the dosage of drugs reduced without sacrificing control of their asthma: a result that could both cut costs for the NHS and reduce side-effects for asthma sufferers. 'A little bit of steroid is good, but if the dose is too high, you get no further benefit and you start to get side-effects. So we performed a large, randomised trial with asthma patients in the community. In one group, we stepped down the dose of inhaled steroids. The other group thought they were having it stepped down, and the investigators thought it was stepped down, but in fact it was staying the same. What we found was that by the end of the study, the step-down group were able to reduce the dose by a significant amount without any loss of asthma control.' This step-down technique is being incorporated into the new national guidelines for asthma management.

In a rather separate area, Thomson and his colleagues are working in collaboration with architects and environmental engineers to investigate whether novel ventilation systems can reduce the level of house dust mites in homes. These mites are one of the commonest allergic triggers of asthma, particularly in children, and it is hoped that this avenue will produce a clinical improvement for patients without the need for drug therapy.

Successful asthma control can only be achieved by using a number of approaches simultaneously, and specialist doctors only provide part of the solution. Other important factors include management of lifestyle and allergic triggers, patient education and access to nurse specialists.

Professor John Warner

There is very little formal provision of hospital allergy services within the NHS, which has made seeing an appropriately trained doctor extremely difficult for many patients, says Professor John Warner, a paediatric allergy specialist at Southampton General Hospital.

'At the moment, allergy services are very poorly distributed and knowledge about allergy is not good, so people are not getting the service that they need and are not receiving a requisite standard of care at all sorts of levels,' he says. 'There are a lot of people ostensibly treating allergic problems and doing it grossly inadequately, without proper training.'

As well as a general shortage of specialist allergy clinics, the service suffers because those that do exist are usually provided on the back of academic departments within university hospitals. Warner says that the allergy service at Southampton General is typical of this. 'The service here is great, but without the academic input it wouldn't exist. If you look around the country, where there are good allergy services they are nearly all allied to academic units and not established services. The worry about that is when, for example, I retire, the next professor of child health may not be interested in allergy, in which case the paediatric allergy service may just disintegrate. When the university advertises, they are not saying we want a paediatric allergist to take over as professor of child health, they want the best academic in any area within paediatrics.'

The lack of formal services in this area means that for parents of children suffering from severe allergies or allergic asthma, finding a doctor at any level of care with an interest in the area can be more productive than a standard referral to the local hospital. 'Some GPs have extensive knowledge of the management of asthma and allergic diseases,' he says. 'They are much better than hospital consultants in general medicine or general paediatrics at managing those diseases, and therefore they can manage severe diseases in primary care. And so be it: they are doing it effectively, they are doing it to a very high standard.'

The problem for parents, then, is finding a doctor locally who is up-to-date in allergy care. Warner thinks that the best way to achieve this is to check with the British Society for Allergy and Clinical Immunology (BSACI), which is the major professional body in the area. 'The BSACI have a list of the GPs who are members,' he says. 'If they are members of that society, you would know, for instance, that at least they are getting a regular journal which tells them what the latest advances are and the opportunity to go to annual meetings to get more information about the leading edge of allergy.'

Warner's own career has been at the frontline of allergy research. He held a clinic for children's allergies at the first dedicated allergy centre in the world, established by Dr John Freeman at St Mary's Hospital in London early in the twentieth century. The main focus of his academic work has been on the origins of allergic disease. 'I have become progressively more involved in trying to identify the early-life origins of allergy, because it has become very apparent that once allergic disease has become established it is very difficult, if not impossible, to switch off,' he says.

Initially, Warner and his colleagues looked for the origins of allergy in children, but they became aware that many of the factors predisposing a person to developing an allergy act much earlier in life. 'It is quite clear that a lot of the seeds of allergic disease are sown very early in pregnancy – during the second trimester,' he says. 'The foetus is already primed immunologically to be more likely to develop allergic disease that early.'

This discovery casts doubt on the prevailing theory that allergies are brought on by lack of childhood exposure to common bacteria in our over-hygienic modern homes – the so-called 'grime hypothesis'. While excessive cleanliness is likely to contribute to allergy development, Warner now believes that there are many other factors as well. 'There are things such as nutrition, which may be very important, the way in which the foetus grows in the womb, and the nutrient delivery that it receives from its mother at various critical stages during development can have profound effects on the way the immune system develops. If people just focus on hygiene they will be forgetting other important factors,' he says.

Both our genes and environment are likely to influence whether we develop allergies, and the precise way in which they act probably varies from person to person. By studying their origins, it may be possible one day to identify and stop allergies from arising in the first place. But even now there are many good treatments available to alleviate suffering and maintain good health. These treatments, however, cannot be used to their full potential in the UK without better training for doctors and a more structured approach to allergy services in general.

Cancer

Although we tend to refer to cancer as if it were a single illness, there are more than 200 different forms. In this section we examine cancer treatment in the UK by looking specifically at two common cancers – breast cancer and colorectal (bowel) cancer. Over the past few years breast cancer survival has increased largely due to increased investment, which has led to better detection as a result of the introduction of a national screening programme and earlier treatment. Bowel cancer, by comparison, although the third most commonly diagnosed cancer in the UK and second most common cause of cancer death, attracts far less investment. The five-year survival rate for colorectal cancer in the UK is lower than in both Europe and the USA. Although the disease is curable in nine out of ten cases if caught early, currently only four out of ten people (40.9 per cent) in the UK survive for longer than five years – 6 per cent fewer than in Europe and 22 per cent fewer than in the USA. Despite the fact that the Government itself estimates that deaths from bowel cancer could fall by 15 per cent if screening were to be introduced, unlike with breast cancer there is no national screening programme. The National Institute for Clinical Excellence (NICE)'s recent decision to limit access to three drugs for advanced colorectal cancer (see p.88) has also been criticised by cancer doctors, who believe more widespread use of the drugs would save lives.

What is the specialty?
This will depend on the type of cancer, but is likely to include: clinical oncology (oncology is the study of cancer) – treatment of cancer with drugs; medical oncology – treatment of cancer with radiotherapy (also called radiology); and surgery. A number of new sub-specialties are emerging, such as colorectal surgery and breast cancer surgery.

What is cancer?
Cancer is a disease of the cells that happens when the cells in a particular part of the body begin to multiply uncontrollably and form a lump or tumour. Tumours may be either malignant (cancerous) or

benign (harmless). The key characteristic of malignant tumours is that, left untreated, they have the ability to invade surrounding tissue and to spread or metastasise to other parts of the body.

What are the statistics?

One in three people in the UK will be diagnosed with some form of cancer in their lifetime and one in four will die from it. Although younger people can get cancer, the disease mainly affects older people, with 65 per cent of cases affecting people aged over 65.

Bowel cancer

Some 18,000 men and 16,000 women in the UK are diagnosed with bowel cancer each year. These statistics make the disease the third most commonly diagnosed cancer in men and the second most commonly diagnosed cancer in women. Bowel cancer is also the second most common cause of overall cancer death (after lung cancer). The disease can affect anyone of any age. However, nine out of ten of those who develop it are aged over 50. The UK has some of the worst survival rates for bowel cancer in the developed world. At best, the rates are comparable with eastern Europe.

Breast cancer

One in nine women will develop breast cancer at some time in their lives and, with approximately 30,000 women being diagnosed with the disease each year and 13,000 dying from it, it is the most common cancer to affect women. Although breast cancer is predominantly a female cancer, a small number of men (around 200) develop the disease each year. The good news is that in recent years there has been a steep decrease in deaths from breast cancer; from 415 for every million of the population in 1986 to 331 per million in 1995. The decline is thought to be in part attributable to greater awareness of symptoms, the introduction of the national breast screening programme for women over 50 and the introduction of new forms of treatment such as tamoxifen (see p.87).

How is it currently treated?

Cancer has been known since ancient times. Indeed, Egyptian papyrus manuscripts record cases of breast tumours, and cancers of the nose and pharynx have been found in Egyptian mummies. The ancient Greeks were the first to recognise cancer as a disease in its own right and to coin the term 'carcinoma' (meaning crab) which is still used today to describe certain kinds of tumour. Ancient Greek statues show ulcerating breast tumours. In fact, mastectomy is one of the oldest operations known. In both ancient Greece and ancient India breast cancers were removed surgically and the wound was treated with herbal poisons in an echo of today's chemotherapy. By the fourteenth century, breast tumours were being treated by blood-sucking leeches and frogs. However, surgery for obviously visible cancers such as those of the breast continued to dominate cancer treatment right up to the twentieth century, with the development of chemotherapy (drug treatment) and radiotherapy. Today, treatments for cancer usually involve one or more of the following.

Surgery

Surgical removal of the tumour in an operation. Solid tumours, such as those of the breast and bowel, will usually involve some kind of surgery.

Chemotherapy

Treatment of the tumour with a number of different types of drugs. This may sometimes be given before surgery – for example, in breast cancer to shrink down the tumour to a state where it is more operable. However, it is most often prescribed after surgery to catch any further cancer cells that might have been difficult to detect, and especially when cancer has been found in nearby lymph nodes, a sign that it has begun to spread.

Radiotherapy

Treatment of the tumour or of residual cancer cells following surgery by high doses of radiation designed to kill any remaining cancer cells and prevent them from spreading.

When chemotherapy and/or radiotherapy are given following surgery this is known as adjuvant therapy.

BOWEL CANCER

The precise treatment offered will depend on the location of the tumour, its size, its stage and whether it has begun to spread.

Surgery is the most common and often the only treatment needed for colorectal cancer, provided it is at an early stage and has not begun to spread. One technique for removing cancers shown to greatly reduce the risk of local recurrence is total mesorectal excision (TME). This involves painstaking dissection and removal of the entire cancer and surrounding tissues so that no satellites remain to spread at a later date. The removed section is checked after the operation to ensure that the entire growth has been taken out (see Heald, p.105). The surgeon will join the bowel back together after a section has been removed. If the tumour is in the lower colon or rectum and the bowel cannot be joined together again, you may need a temporary or permanent colostomy or ileostomy procedure, in which the opening of the bowel (stoma) is rerouted on to the skin of the abdominal wall, enabling faeces to be collected in a bag.

Chemotherapy may be given before or after surgical removal of the tumour. The most common chemotherapy drug for colorectal cancer is 5-fluorouracil (5-FU), usually given in combination with a vitamin called folinic acid. Radiotherapy is most often used to treat cancer of the rectum, but is not usually used for cancer of the colon.

Surgery may also be used in more advanced bowel cancer to remove bowel obstruction. However, once cancer has spread beyond the bowel the most usual treatment is chemotherapy.

BREAST CANCER

Breast cancer is treated with surgery, radiotherapy, chemotherapy and hormonal therapy. The precise mix of these therapies will depend on many different factors, such as your age, the position, size and type of your cancer and whether it has spread. Because there is no clear-cut 'best' treatment for breast cancer, the doctor will want to involve you closely to ensure any treatment decisions are right for you.

Surgery for breast cancer may involve either a lumpectomy (wide local excision), in which the tumour and a small part of the surrounding tissue is removed, or a mastectomy, in which the whole breast is removed.

If you have a mastectomy, you may be offered breast reconstruction – either immediate or delayed – to give a breast shape. There are several different options available.

If you decide to have a lumpectomy, you will be offered radiotherapy to eliminate any residual cancer cells. Radiotherapy may be offered after a total mastectomy to destroy any residual cancer cells. Radiotherapy may be given externally or internally by inserting wires containing a radioactive substance into the breast to provide a dose of radiotherapy to the breast tissue.

The doctor will also take a few glands from your armpit (axillary nodes) to check if the cancer has begun to spread, a procedure called axillary node sampling. If there are any cancer cells in the axillary nodes, the doctor may remove all the lymph glands under your arm (axillary clearance) or offer radiotherapy.

Chemotherapy may be given before surgery (neoadjuvant chemotherapy) or, more conventionally, after surgery to destroy any remaining cancer cells. Typically this involves giving a cocktail of three drugs, for example, cyclophosphamide, methotrexate and 5-fluorouracil (CMF).

Pre-menopausal women undergoing surgery or investigation for breast cancer may have dramatically improved survival rates if they are treated in the second half of their menstrual cycle, according to research conducted by Professor Ian Fentiman (see p.102); however, the idea that the timing of surgery has an effect on outcomes in breast cancer remains controversial.

The big revolution in breast cancer treatment came with the introduction of tamoxifen, a hormonal drug, which may be given alone or in combination with chemotherapy. Today, a number of hormonal therapies are available, all with slightly different modes of action. Tamoxifen is particularly effective in post-menopausal women with tumours that are fuelled by the female sex hormone oestrogen. This is referred to as being oestrogen-receptor positive or HER2 positive. In pre-menopausal women, removal of the ovaries (ablation), either surgically, chemically or with radiotherapy, lowers oestrogen levels and can reduce the risk of recurrence. A number of drugs can also be used that stop the ovaries from functioning.

How does that measure up to treatment in the rest of Europe and the USA?

Compared to the rest of Europe, the UK has abysmally low rates for survival from bowel cancer, although breast cancer survival rates are rising. This can be attributed to a shortage of specialised cancer doctors (see Cassidy, p.98), fewer radiotherapy machines and equipment, fewer specialist nurses, and difficulty in getting modern chemotherapy treatments licensed and approved.

To take just one example, combination therapy with the new chemotherapy drugs irinotecan (Campto) or oxaliplatin (Eloxatin) with 5-fluoracil, a recognised treatment for early bowel cancer in Europe, is not able to be prescribed in the UK because NICE has failed to approve it for this purpose. Another problem is the length of time taken for the approval process for new drugs. All new drugs have to go through separate national pricing and reimbursement negotiations, which can in some cases take years. In the UK, for example, the drug docetaxel (Taxotere), which is used to treat advanced breast cancer, took four -and -a -half years from initial approval by the European Medicines Evaluation Agency to approval by NICE.

There are huge differences between cancer outcomes in the UK and the USA too. Although the basic treatments of surgery, chemotherapy and radiotherapy remain the same, the USA tends to get there first with new developments in treatment, such as new drugs. The USA also recommends regular screening for bowel cancer, and breast cancer screening starts earlier there – at 40 rather than 50 in the UK. Doctors tend to treat both bowel and breast cancer more aggressively at an earlier stage than they do here.

What new treatments are available?

Breast cancer

A number of new drug treatments have become available in the past few years. These include taxanes for the treatment of advanced breast cancer and trastuzumab (Herceptin), a new type of anti-cancer drug called a monoclonal antibody, that works by blocking the access of HER2, which fuels the growth of breast cancer, by locking on to receptors on breast cancer cells and blocking their growth (rather like a key fitting into a lock).

Bowel cancer

As well as the two new drugs mentioned above, there is also an oral form of 5-FU, capecitabine (Xeloda), which is said to be safer and less toxic than the traditional version, which has to be injected.

Can I get these on the NHS?

In the past year, NICE has issued guidelines on the use of the monoclonal antibody treatment Herceptin (see above) for the treatment of advanced breast cancer. However, patients in the UK have had to wait a long time for a drug that has been widely prescribed in the USA and Europe for some time now, and even today some women face problems in getting treatment.

In March 2002, following a successful appeal by CancerBACUP, NICE decided that one of the new bowel cancer therapies, oxaliplatin (Eloxatin) could be prescribed for bowel cancer sufferers with potentially operable secondary liver tumours. However, many, including CancerBACUP itself, argue that the NICE decision didn't go far enough. Patients who can't tolerate oxaliplatin have no choice but to pay out of their own pockets if they want one of the other modern chemotherapy treatments for bowel cancer, such as irinotecan (Campto). What's more, NICE also ruled against the routine prescription of the two drugs in combination with 5-FU for people with early bowel cancer (see p.88).

It's the same story with capecitabine (see p.88). Despite large-scale randomised trials showing its safety and efficacy, the drug is currently available only in the private sector.

What treatments are in the pipeline?

There is a clutch of new drugs in the pipeline. These include drugs designed to counteract cancer by cutting off the tumour's blood supply, and EGF (epidermal growth factor) inhibitors that work by interfering with the ability of cancer cells to grow uncontrollably at the same time as enhancing the power of chemotherapy.

In one approach, a vaccine is being developed against a receptor molecule found on the surface of some cancer cells. The injected vaccine consists of DNA, which is taken up by the body cells and used to make a protein. The protein produced triggers a reaction from the patient's immune system that it is hoped will destroy the cancer (see Coombes, p.101).

In breast cancer, new hormonal drugs are being developed, such as fulvestrant (Faslodex), a new anti-oestrogen hormonal drug, which has fewer side-effects than the ones currently used. Mastectomy also seems to be becoming slightly more popular as an option, with new methods of breast reconstruction being pioneered by surgeons in some hospitals.

Bowel cancer too is seeing an explosion of potential new approaches.

- **New combination therapies:** the large FOCUS trial being mounted by the Medical Research Council is looking at whether treatment with a combination of the two chemotherapy drugs irnotecan and oxaliplatin slows progression of advanced colon cancer. Scientists are also examining whether it is preferable to give either of the two drugs together with the more usual standard treatment, 5-FU (known as combination therapy), as a first treatment or only if the cancer spreads after treatment with 5-FU.
- **Bowel cancer vaccine:** trials of a bowel cancer vaccine are under way to see if giving the vaccine before or after surgery reduces the risk of recurrence.
- **Bowel cancer screening:** the Government is currently piloting a two-year colorectal screening programme for people aged between 50 and 69 to see whether testing for hidden blood in the stools (faecal occult blood) saves lives. People registered with a GP in a number of sites throughout the UK will be offered a faecal occult blood test (FOBT) to screen for bowel cancer. It's estimated that screening could save the lives of 2,500 people a year.

Who treats it?

Clinical oncologist: a specialist in cancer treatment with drugs.

Surgeon: a specialist with training in surgery. In the case of breast cancer you should ideally have a specialist breast surgeon. If you are having reconstruction, it's particularly important to see a surgeon who is experienced in performing this procedure. In the case of bowel surgery, there are consultants who specialise in this form of surgery.

Medical oncologist (radiologist): a specialist in treatment using radiotherapy.

What training will the specialist(s) have?

Before becoming a consultant, your doctor will have had a general medical training, which includes five years at university followed by one year as a House Officer, before gaining registration with the General Medical Council. They will then have spent two to three years as a Senior House Officer in various medical disciplines. This is followed by a five- or six-year period of specialist registrar training, working in different hospitals, leading to a Certificate of Completion of Specialist Training that is recognised throughout Europe. In the fifth year and post-certification, doctors are encouraged to train to become sub-specialists.

An increasing number of consultants will now be specifically trained in, say, bowel cancer surgery or breast reconstructive surgery. For many patients, the most important factor in beating cancer will be the skill of their surgeon (Monson, p.108).

Where will I receive care?

If you are diagnosed with cancer, you may be treated in your local hospital. Many people with cancer will see the specialist at one of the 34 cancer centres based in large general hospitals throughout England and Wales. You should see the whole multi-disciplinary team when you are first diagnosed and should see the individual specialist before and during the various forms of treatment. The specialist or a member of his/her team should also see you when you attend for follow-up.

What questions should I ask about my treatment?

- What is the usual treatment for this kind of cancer?
- Will I be offered chemotherapy before surgery or after surgery?
- Will I need radiotherapy?
- Why is chemotherapy recommended at this time?
- Are there any other options?
- What is the chance of recurrence?
- How will I know if my cancer has recurred?
- How many courses of chemotherapy will I need?
- How long will treatment last?
- What drugs will be used?
- How will they be administered?
- What side-effects can I expect?
- What can be done to alleviate side-effects?
- Are there any clinical trials being performed that could help me?
- Will treatment affect my fertility?
- What can I do to help myself?
- How often will I have to attend for check-ups?
- Will I have to attend for check-ups for the rest of my life?

Women

- Will I be able to get pregnant?
- How soon after treatment may I start trying to conceive?
- Will treatment bring on an early menopause?

What will my treatment involve?

Initial treatment

If you are advised to have surgery you will have to spend some time in hospital. External radiotherapy is usually done on an outpatient basis, and you will have to attend for a detailed planning appointment to assess what is needed and exactly where the radiotherapy should be delivered, followed by daily attendance over a period of several weeks. If you are having internal radiotherapy this will usually be done in hospital.

You will also have to attend the hospital for chemotherapy. Depending on the way the drugs are administered, this may include hospital stays of a day or two. Some chemotherapy drugs are tablets, but many are injected or dripped (infused) into a vein. You will also have to attend the hospital for regular check-ups such as blood tests, scans and other tests to monitor your response. The usual regimen involves a course of drugs followed by a rest to allow your body time to recover, usually around six months.

Side-effects

Both radiotherapy and drug treatments can cause side-effects. The precise ones you experience will depend on the treatment, the dosage and how the drugs used affect you personally. No two people react in exactly the same way. Some common side-effects include nausea and vomiting, hair loss and an increased tendency to develop infections caused by chemotherapy drugs affecting the body's white blood cell count. Lymphoedema, a collection of fluid caused by damage to the lymphatic system, is another potential complication of surgery and radiotherapy. The specialist cancer nurse can talk to you about what side-effects you may experience and how to deal with them.

Follow-up

Once your cancer has gone into remission, you will have to attend outpatient clinics at regular intervals to check that you are well and that there is no recurrence. At first, these check-ups will be at short intervals of three and six months. However, as time goes on they will gradually become less frequent – usually annual. In some units the specialist may sign you off altogether after a variable period of between five and ten years.

What makes a REAL difference to getting better?

- **Early diagnosis.** Getting a diagnosis at a point when a cancer is in an early treatable form is crucial for many different forms of cancer. This applies to both breast and bowel cancer. Survival rates from breast cancer have increased since the introduction of the Government's national breast screening programme, which offers women aged 50 to 64 the chance to have three-yearly mammographic screening, and this is thought to be one factor (along with greater awareness and the availability of more effective drugs) in the drop in breast cancer deaths that has been seen recently.

Research shows that having your treatment supervised by a multi-disciplinary team that includes specialist doctors, nurses and other healthcare professionals offers the best chance of recovery (see Coombes, p.101).

- **Innovative treatments.** Treatment for cancer is extremely complex, and the exact treatment you need will be highly individual. In the case of breast cancer, for example, the introduction of hormonal therapies such as tamoxifen has contributed to the improvement in survival rates, transforming the disease from one that women almost inevitably died from to one that many live with for long periods of time.

A survey of cancer specialists carried out in 2001 by the Cancer Research Campaign (now part of Cancer Research UK) found that doctors blamed lack of access to innovative chemotherapy treatments as the main factor in the poor management of bowel cancer in the UK. Research also shows that people who enter clinical trials of new drugs and treatments do better on average than those who receive standard treatment.

What is the difference between a well-run and a badly run cancer service?

The biggest difference is the availability of a multi-disciplinary team, who hold regular meetings to discuss your case, so you can be sure that your care and treatment are coordinated and consistent (see

Coombes, p.101). Many excellent cancer services are provided out of buildings that are not modern. However, ideally a well-run service should have some or all of the following features:

Services all in one place

In many hospitals you have to trail all over the hospital for different services. For example, you may have to go to radiology for X-rays, ultrasound, mammograms and other types of scanning, to the pathology department for blood tests and then to yet another part of the hospital to see the oncologist or surgeon. Ideally, all cancer services should be under the same roof and in the same place.

Dedicated waiting area

In many hospitals you have to wait in a general outpatient department, with patients waiting for other conditions to be diagnosed or treated, rather than in a specific cancer waiting area. It's less stressful for everyone concerned if the unit has its own dedicated waiting area.

Dedicated cancer clinics

Dedicated clinics where people with suspected cancer can be seen are also part of a well-run service. In some hospitals, women waiting for a diagnosis of breast cancer may be waiting with women with benign breast conditions.

Privacy

Being told you have cancer is a stressful experience. In a well-run clinic there should be provision for you to receive your diagnosis in a private place and to have somewhere private where you can go afterwards to talk to your partner or companion.

Access to a specialist nurse and other specific services

Support and access to accurate, high-quality information are important aspects of cancer care. For example, the clinic should have a breast care nurse(s) or bowel nurse specialist(s) who will accompany you when you receive your diagnosis and who will be available for you and/or your family to talk to if you have any worries. Other services specific to your particular kind of cancer should also be provided; for example, prosthesis and bra-fitting for women who have had a mastectomy, or specialist advice on colostomy for people who have had this procedure.

Will I get better treatment if I go privately?

You may well have access to some of the newer drugs and treatments if you choose to go privately. The 'hotel' side of your care – the hospital environment, your room, meals and services such as telephone or television – will almost certainly be better too, and the surgeon will usually have longer to spend with you. On the other hand, most specialists who work privately also do NHS work, so you may well see exactly the same specialist as you would have done on the NHS. You will also have access to clinical trials if you go on the NHS. Another point to bear in mind is that many private hospitals have no medical staff on duty at night, so you may well be better off in an NHS hospital where there is medical back-up if needed. The key is to be treated by a specialised, multi-disciplinary team.

Will I get better treatment if I go abroad?

According to a new law, anyone now has the right to seek treatment in the European Union on the NHS if there is an excessive wait here or if there is good reason why you should have a particular 'well-established' treatment not available here. It's worth bearing in mind, however, that if you are hoping to be paid for by the NHS, your consultant must agree that treatment is necessary and can only be obtained abroad. The NHS will pay only for evidence-based treatments and not for trial drugs or experimental therapies. So unless you can afford to pay (and most new cancer drugs and procedures are expensive), you won't have access to them. You also need to consider the potential stress of travelling, of language difficulties and of being far from family and friends.

What support will I be offered by the clinic and are there any independent support groups I can join?

You should have the support of a specialist cancer nurse, whom you can ring at any time with any problems or worries you may have. Some units have special support groups for patients with specific types of cancer who have been treated there. The specialist cancer nurse will usually be able to give you useful leaflets, and some units may have a library in-site with useful books, videos and publications that you can borrow. The unit should also be able to put you in touch with the local branches of any relevant cancer support groups.

Useful addresses

GENERAL CANCER
Cancer BACUP
3 Bath Place
Rivington Street
London EC2A 3JR
Tel 020 7613 2121
Freephone 0808 800 1234 (9 am to 7 pm Monday to Friday)
www.cancerbacup.org.uk

Cancer Care Society
11 The Cornmarket
Romsey
Hampshire SO51 8GB
Tel 01794 830300
www.cancercaresoc.demon.co.uk

Macmillan Cancer Relief
(Merged with Cancerlink)
89 Albert Embankment
London SE1 7UQ
Tel 020 7840 7840
Helpline 0808 808000
www.cancerlink.org

BREAST CANCER
Breast Cancer Care
Kiln House
210 New King's Road
London SW6 4NZ
Tel 020 7384 2984
Helpline 0808 800 6000 (10 am to 5 pm Monday to Friday,
10 am to 2 pm Saturday)
www.breastcancercare.org.uk

UK Breast Cancer Coalition

Suite 1D, Broadway House

112–134 The Broadway

London SW19 1RL

Tel 020 8543 4455

www.ukbcc.org.uk

BOWEL CANCER

Beating Bowel Cancer

39 Crown Road

St Margarets

Twickenham TW1 3EJ

Tel 020 8892 5256

www.beatingbowelcancer.org

The Bowel Cancer Forum

An umbrella organisation that includes ten separate charities

www.bowelcancerforum.co.uk

Colon Cancer Concern

9 Rickett Street

London SW6 1RU

Tel 020 7381 9711

Infoline 08708 506050 (10 am to 4 pm Monday to Friday)

www.coloncancer.org.uk

Pelican Cancer Foundation

North Hampshire Hospital

Aldermarston Road

Basingstoke

Hampshire RG24 9NA

www.pelicancentre.com/charity.html

Expert opinions

Professor Jim Cassidy

Over a quarter of Scottish colon cancer patients never get to see a specialist oncologist, denying them access to an increasingly effective range of cancer drugs for treating the condition and preventing its recurrence, says Professor Jim Cassidy, head of the Beatson Oncology Centre in Glasgow, which is Scotland's largest cancer treatment facility. 'This is a very important issue, and something that this country urgently needs to turn around,' he says. 'People must be made to think, "Hey, wait a minute, I've got cancer. I should be seeing someone who has got oncology written on their badge."'

The problem is partly a historical one. Colon cancer has long been considered one of the forms of the disease that is most resistant to chemotherapy treatment. 'Colon cancer was one of a number of diseases in which medical oncology and chemotherapy were not particularly used. That was what interested me about it in the first place,' he says.

In the last ten years, however, both the chemotherapy drugs and the systems for delivering them to where they are needed in the body have improved, and oncologists are now able to do much more for patients suffering from colon cancer. The problem now is actually getting to see an oncologist, and Cassidy's advice is to be firm. 'The patient or the patient's GP has got to push really hard and not be put off or deflected away from the idea. There are many people who will say, "You don't need to see an oncologist because they won't do anything for you," or alternatively, "Oh, they're really bad people and they will poison you with nasty drugs." It is not right. It's like me trying to give someone advice on whether they should have an operation or not. I wouldn't dare to do that. We would send them to the surgeon and let the surgeon decide what's best.'

Lack of access to specialist oncology has not been the only problem facing Scotland's cancer patients in the last few years. Before Cassidy took over in February 2002, the Beatson had suffered a long series of problems, including low staff morale, underfunding, and long waiting times, and the Government is now committed to building a brand new centre to replace the existing buildings.

While this will alleviate some of the problems, Cassidy feels that more effort should be made to educate people in Glasgow's poorer communities about their healthcare options. 'Here is Glasgow, we have more social deprivation than you could shake a stick at, and most of the patients who come from that segment of the community have almost no concept of healthcare at all,' says Cassidy. 'You almost have to start from scratch with them. We try to make up the information deficit, but in terms of getting the best out of the system, they certainly don't ask the questions they should of their consultants. These are questions like, "What are your qualifications for doing this?" or "How many patients do you see per month?" or "What are your success rates?" People are either unaware, reticent or embarrassed about asking these questions.'

Cassidy has also been involved in a study comparing the ways in which people from rural areas access cancer services relative to those from cities. This has also revealed deficits in education. 'There was a difference for patients from country areas, but it was probably not the medical services that failed them. Rather, they themselves tended to hold on to their symptoms for longer before they went to their GP. So there is an educational argument there about how you could teach people in the country to be more aware of healthcare issues.'

Only with more emphasis on education will people from deprived or rural areas be empowered to ask the right questions and influence the direction of their care. And as the current crisis in access to oncology services illustrates, this kind of initiative is badly needed.

Professor Charles Coombes

Some oncologists are failing to keep up with advances in the treatment of individual cancers because they are seeing patients with too many different forms of the disease, says Professor Charles Coombes, a world leading expert in the treatment of advanced breast cancer and head of the cancer studies research group at Imperial College in London. He feels that oncologists should limit themselves to a maximum of two different types of cancer.

'The first thing for patients to find out is how many other types of cancer does their doctor treat, because if it is more than two you can be pretty sure that he or she is not keeping up with modern practice,' he says. 'Two types of cancer is the maximum anyone can realistically be expected to keep up with at the moment. They won't have time to attend the multi-disciplinary meetings or go to the international meetings if they are doing more than two.'

The number of cancer patients who see an oncologist has increased dramatically in recent years, and the complexity of the treatments available has also risen. The resultant rise in the oncology workload has not been matched by a sufficient increase in the number of doctors, which contributes to the problem of individual consultants seeing too many forms of cancer. 'Twenty years ago, maybe one patient in ten with breast cancer had chemotherapy, whereas now I would say it is nearer six out of ten,' says Coombes. 'Whereas the rest of Europe and North America recognised the need and kept up with requirements, this country has not.'

Spiralling workloads also impact on whether consultants have time for research. And while some good oncologists do not contribute to a lot of papers, those that do are likely to be up- to-date in the field. Patients can easily check a doctor's research record on the internet, and Coombes thinks that this is a useful thing to do. 'Most oncologists should be getting their names onto some papers,' he says. 'It's very simple for patients to find out just by looking on the internet under Pub Med and typing the doctor's name and the subject. If they are not engaged in any research in a fast-moving area like cancer, I would be slightly concerned.'

The emphasis in modern breast cancer care is on a multi-disciplinary approach, which means that the oncologists work closely with other professionals such as surgeons and specialist nurses. Coombes believes that patients should also be wary of a breast cancer service that is not constituted in this way. 'If it is a sole consultant, with nobody around him or her, then I think that is telling you all sorts of things,' he says. 'It usually means that the consultant has not made the effort to get people, and the consultants who can't be bothered to put in a business case for obviously required staff are also the ones who can't be bothered to check whether they are giving up-to-date, modern advice.'

Similarly, if the service does not have a one-stop breast clinic, where diagnostic tests are performed and the results returned on the same day, there is something seriously wrong, he says.

Coombes is the director of one of the largest cancer research laboratories in the country, with around 120 doctors and scientists studying ways to improve the effectiveness of the drugs used to treat cancer. 'Most current chemotherapy drugs kill cancer cells by interfering with their DNA, which is a broad-spectrum, blunderbuss approach,' he says. 'However, things are improving since we can now identify molecular targets associated with breast cancer, which we then engineer treatments for.'

In one approach, they are developing a vaccine against a receptor molecule found on the surface of some cancer cells. The injected vaccine consists of DNA, which is taken up by the body cells and used to make a protein. The protein produced triggers a reaction from the patient's immune system that it is hoped will destroy the cancer.

New approaches like this are still some way from becoming effective treatments, but this is an extremely active area of research, with new therapies becoming available all the time.

Professor Ian Fentiman

Major steps are needed to introduce more flexibility in the timing of operations and to combat ageism if death rates from breast cancer are to improve, says a leading expert in the condition.

Pre-menopausal women undergoing surgery or investigation for breast cancer have dramatically improved survival rates if they are treated in the second half of their menstrual cycle, according to research conducted by Professor Ian Fentiman, a consultant surgeon at the Guy's Hospital clinical oncology unit in London. However, this simple and potentially life-saving observation has not been put into practice at many of the country's cancer units.

'It is difficult to believe that it's actually 11 years ago that we first published this in the *Lancet*,' says Fentiman. 'But it seems that people are very reluctant to do something so simple as changing the time of surgery, and so in most places it doesn't happen. When you look at the figures involved, I would have said that since 1991, if people had changed their timing, it would have saved 2,000 or 3,000 lives.'

The Guy's results are certainly dramatic. Researchers looked back over many years at the records of patients who had undergone surgery at the unit for breast cancer that had spread to the lymph glands. They found substantial differences between those who were operated on in the first half of the menstrual cycle (the follicular phase) and those who were treated in the second half (the luteal phase). 'To put figures on this, if you have a group of women having surgery in the luteal phase of the cycle, after ten years 78 per cent of them will be alive. If you look at women who have had surgery in the follicular phase, at ten years 33 per cent of them will be alive. It is such a large difference, bigger than any form of adjuvant treatment ever used.'

The effect is not limited to surgery. Fentiman and his colleagues also found a link between the timing of a diagnostic procedure called core biopsy, in which a large needle is used to extract a sample of breast tissue for analysis, and the risk of the cancer recurring. Again, having the investigation in the early part of the cycle, when levels of oestrogen (a hormone implicated in the growth of some breast cancers) are at their highest, resulted in worse outcomes.

'Some women who had been operated on in the second half of the cycle had needle biopsies in the first half,' he says. 'This was a relatively small group, around eight to ten of them, but we found that all of those individuals had a recurrance within two years. What this was saying was that the very act of doing a needle biopsy was actually shedding cells which were going to other parts of the body. This was happening at a time when there were oestrogens around, which enabled them to establish themselves.'

The idea that the timing of surgery has an effect on outcomes in breast cancer is controversial. And there have been some studies performed subsequently that have not agreed with Fentiman's conclusions. However, he is keen to emphasise that analyses undertaken elsewhere using all the available data have found that there is an effect.

For patients awaiting breast surgery or needle biopsy who are concerned about the timing of their treatment, Fentiman's advice is not to be pushed around. 'I've had a lot of people ring me up and ask what they should do. The answer is that you can turn around and say, "Look, you may not believe it, but I believe it and could you please book me in for a particular time." There should be enough leeway in the system such that if a patient says they want to have their operation done at a particular time, they actually can have it done at that time.'

While getting the timing of treatment right is a problem for pre-menopausal women, Fentiman feels that it is the older women with breast cancer who are really missing out on the best-quality care. 'We have a lot of evidence, not just from Britain but from all over the world, that women over the age of 70 are inadequately treated much of the time,' he says. 'When you consider that the average life expectancy of a woman of 70 in Britain is 15 years, if you mistreat her breast cancer or under-treat it, she will live long enough for that cancer to come back and possibly kill her prematurely.'

There are several key areas in which elderly women with breast cancer are under-treated on the NHS. First, the breast screening programme, even when its upper age limit is extended to 69 next year, will still exclude women of 70 or over – a group that accounts for 40 per cent of all cases of the disease. Without screening, older women with breast cancer tend to be picked up later, and sometimes a decision is made not to treat them in the standard way. Examples of this include reduced use of breast-conserving surgical techniques, based on a false premise that older women are less concerned about losing a breast, or even a refusal to consider surgery at all. 'There are still quite a lot of people who, if they have got an older woman with breast cancer, just give her tamoxifen, and we know that is not an adequate method of treatment. If the woman is going to be living for more than a year – in other words, if she doesn't have other serious diseases – she is going to be at a very high risk of a recurrence.'

Fentiman feels that older patients are neglected in part because of a prevailing attitude among their generation that makes them less inclined to question their treatment. Some have younger relatives who can help to ensure they are getting appropriate care, but if overall outcomes are to improve, the current inequity in access to treatments will have to be addressed.

Professor Bill Heald

There are large variations in skill and surgical techniques between surgeons operating on cancers of the bowel and rectum, and these factors can greatly influence the risk of surgery failing to cure the disease, says Professor Bill Heald, the Macmillan Professor of Surgery at North Hampshire Hospital in Basingstoke.

Improvements in surgery have made cancers of the colon and rectum among the most curable of all cancers. However, surgery sometimes fails, and the major indicator of this is when the cancer returns after the operation in the same part of the body – an event that doctors call local recurrence. When cancer does return in the same area, the outlook for patients is not good, as treatment options are limited. For this reason, Heald thinks that it is very important for patients with the disease to invest time in finding a good surgeon.

'One of the principal things I would advise the really enquiring patient to do is to find out whether the person they are going to has published their results,' he says. 'Publications in peer-reviewed journals, like *The Lancet*, the *British Journal of Surgery* and so on, would be very high up on my list of how you should judge who are the best guys.'

Where published results are not readily available, Heald's advice is to ask the surgeon directly, though he concedes that patients can find it awkward to ask these questions in a tactful way. In addition to finding out about the surgeon's rate for local recurrences, it is useful to know what percentage of operations result in permanent colostomies, what proportion of patients retain sexual function and whether the surgeon will be involved personally in the operation. 'Operations on rectal cancer should be done with a very senior surgeon present, by which I mean either a consultant or a fifth- or sixth-year specialist registrar,' he says. 'I don't really think that rectal cancer should be regarded any longer as an operation that can be done by an unspecialised trainee.'

Heald's major contribution to colorectal cancer surgery has been in refining and promoting a technique for removing cancers called total mesorectal excision (TME). The operation, which can take up to five hours, involves painstaking dissection and removal of the entire cancer and surrounding tissues so that no satellites remain to spread at a later date. The removed section is checked after the operation to ensure that the entire growth, as well as any stray cells, has been taken out.

The TME technique is becoming more widespread, and as a recent German study indicates, where surgeons have adopted it, has had a significant impact on the rate of local recurrence of these cancers. 'In various German surgeons, all in first-class German hospitals, the local recurrence rate varied from 5 per cent to 55 per cent,' says Heald. 'There is no other form of cancer treatment where the variations are so great, and their perception of the reason was that of the TME technique, which had been introduced in one or two of the hospitals, but not in the others.'

At Heald's own unit in Basingstoke, the local recurrence rate is around 5 per cent, one of the lowest in the world, and a charity called the Pelican Cancer Foundation has been established there to spread the use of TME and other good practice in colorectal surgery to other centres. 'The Foundation is particularly dedicated as a charity to the idea of improving the quality of bowel cancer surgery, and that really has been my life's work,' he says.

The quality of the surgery is not the only factor that patients should look at, as treatments like radiotherapy can also have significant benefits. For radiotherapy to be administered appropriately, however, Heald believes that an MRI scan is necessary to determine the extent of the cancer, and this is not currently carried out at all units. 'Before they go into the operation, patients should have had a fine-slice MRI scan (i.e. a highly detailed scan) to try to decide whether radiotherapy should be given before the operation or whether it is not needed,' he says. 'At the moment, what's happening in a lot of places is that people get radiotherapy anyway and I don't really think that is justified, because long-term there are adverse consequences of radiotherapy, and so you need to be sure.' These consequences can include a deterioration of sexual function and a long-term increased risk of a further cancer developing in the irradiated areas. So it is worth finding out, through charities like Colon Cancer Concern or the Pelican Cancer Foundation itself, which units have modern, fine-slice MRI facilities.

While radiotherapy can be important in reducing the size of tumours prior to surgery, and improved surgical techniques like TME reduce the risk of local recurrence, curing colon cancer remains highly dependent on the skill of the surgeon. Heald feels that the best way for patients to judge this is by looking up their surgeon's published results.

Professor John Monson

For many cancer patients, the most important factor in beating the disease will be finding the right surgeon, according to Professor John Monson, head of the academic surgery unit at Castle Hill Hospital in Hull. 'In the vast majority of the big killing cancers – breast, colorectal, lung, cervical, ovarian and gastrointestinal cancers – survival depends on their stage of diagnosis and their surgical treatment. The bulk of survival in all of these cancers is derived from surgery alone,' he says.

Other forms of treatment, such as chemotherapy and radiotherapy, can deliver great benefits to some, but their overall impact is still less than surgery. 'If one looks at the potential impact on outcomes of chemotherapy in breast cancer or colon cancer, for example, adjuvant chemotherapy probably produces about a 10 to 12 per cent absolute increase in survival, which is an important but relatively modest increase.'

The problem for patients is that surgical skill is extremely difficult for them to assess. Important factors to look at include whether the person they are seeing has a declared special interest in the treatment being proposed and what proportion of their workload is dedicated to the condition. Monson feels that it is advisable to ask about this during the initial consultation. 'If somebody says to me, "Well, you tell me you are a colorectal surgeon, what evidence do you have? Who says you are?" I'm not going to be offended by that question,' he says. 'I think the patient needs to take some responsibility for their own care and not be afraid to ask. If your surgeon is offended by being asked these questions, as a general rule of thumb it's probably not unreasonable to say that you are seeing the wrong person,' he adds.

While most well-trained, competent general surgeons around the country can do routine colon cancer surgery, problems arise when you move beyond the routine into the more complex and difficult cases. Surgeons themselves know that when complications arise, having a real expert in charge can make all the difference. 'If you ask any surgeon – and it's a common question in surgical meetings – which operation would you have for this condition, most surgeons would say that the first question should be that it's not a matter of which operation, it's which surgeon,' he says.

While there is no doubt that finding an expert surgeon can improve outcomes in colon cancer, overall survival rates are heavily dependent on the stage at which the condition is detected. A significant problem in this area is that waiting times for the major diagnostic test for the condition, colonoscopy, are often long. 'There are big problems nationally in terms of waiting times for colonoscopy for all sorts of reasons, one of which is shortage of endoscopists,' says Monson. 'But providing access to early investigation instead of waiting too long makes a big difference. Colon cancer is a condition which if treated in its advanced stage has a very poor prognosis, but if treated in its early stages has a chance of cure in the region of 90 per cent.'

Monson's unit is developing new diagnostic techniques for colon cancer designed to reduce delays in diagnosis. One of the most promising of these is virtual colonoscopy, in which a computerised tomography (CT) scanner is used to provide a detailed picture of the colon without using an endoscope.

'Virtual colonoscopy is a radiological technique that provides a good imaging of the inside of the colon without actually doing a colonoscopy. It uses high-resolution, fast-acting CT scanners and computers to produce a virtual 3-D reconstruction of the colon. It's not totally non-invasive but dramatically less invasive than a full colonoscopy, and it is much quicker and easier to do,' he says. 'It's relatively early in its developmental stages and therefore there isn't very large data out there to say how accurate it is – although what data there is out there suggests that for detecting the lesions that matter it's pretty accurate.'

A less high-tech approach that is already making an impact on colonoscopy waiting times has been the introduction of nurse practitioners trained in flexible sigmoidoscopy, and in this area, too, the Hull unit has taken a lead. 'This unit is responsible for the design and establishment of the national nurse practitioner training course for flexible sigmoidoscopy, and most of the nurse practitioners doing this in the UK were trained in Hull,' he says. 'A flexible sigmoidoscopy, if you like, is a sort of half colonoscopy. It uses a flexible, fibre-optic endoscope, which looks at the left-hand side of the colon, which is the main area of interest in that most of the malignant lesions are in that part of the colon and within reach of that scope.'

Techniques like virtual colonoscopy and flexible sigmoidoscopy will probably help doctors to catch colon cancer earlier in the future, so outcomes can be expected to improve. However, skilful surgery still offers the best chance of beating the disease. And with degrees of experience in the condition varying widely between surgeons, it is important for patients to check for themselves that the person they are seeing has the required expertise.

Diabetes

What is the specialty?

It varies, but it may be general medicine, endocrinology (the study of hormones) or diabetology (the study of diabetes mellitus).

What is diabetes?

Diabetes is a condition in which the amount of glucose in the blood is too high because the pancreas does not make enough insulin, or the insulin produced is ineffective, or a combination of both. Insulin is the hormone responsible for helping glucose (sugar) from the digestion of carbohydrate in food move into the body's cells, where it is used for energy. When insulin is not present or is ineffective, glucose builds up in the blood. There are two main types of diabetes.

TYPE 1 DIABETES (insulin-dependent diabetes)

This typically develops before the age of 40 (often, although not always, during childhood and adolescence). Type 1 diabetes is an autoimmune condition, in which the immune system turns against and destroys the islets of Langerhans – the beta cells of the pancreas that produce insulin. This results in a complete absence of insulin.

TYPE 2 DIABETES

This tends to occur after the age of 40, although it may appear earlier in people of South Asian and African-Caribbean origin. It is caused either by a shortage of insulin or by the body developing an inability to use insulin properly, known as insulin resistance. Although the condition is often referred to as noninsulin-dependent diabetes, this is not strictly accurate, as Type 2 diabetes is a progressive condition and a number of people with it do end up having to inject insulin. Type 2 diabetes is more common than Type 1 and affects over 80 per cent of the total number of people with diabetes.

There are also several other, rarer, types of diabetes, including gestational diabetes, which appears during pregnancy, and maturity onset diabetes of the young (MODY).

What are the statistics?

Diabetes is one of the most common conditions of the endocrine (hormonal) system all over the world and in every age group. Worldwide, the condition is sharply on the increase, and in the UK 1.4 million people have been diagnosed with diabetes, while a further million are thought to have it without knowing it (see Barnett, p.123).

Diabetes affects men and women equally, but is three to five times more common among people of African-Caribbean and South Asian background. Diabetes is not just serious in itself but can cause serious complications as well. Up to seven out of ten people with Type 2 diabetes have high blood pressure and a similar number have raised cholesterol levels, both of which increase the risk of developing heart disease. There is also a risk of other complications caused by damage to the eyes (diabetic retinopathy), kidneys (diabetic nephropathy), nerves (diabetic neuropathy), heart and blood vessels (cardiovascular complications). Diabetes is said to account for some 9 per cent of the annual NHS budget (see Barnett, p.123).

How is it currently treated?

Diabetes has been known since ancient times, but it was not until the nineteenth century that it began to be understood as originating in the pancreas. The first big breakthrough in treatment came with the discovery of insulin at the University of Toronto in 1921. Before that, the only way to manage diabetes was to go on a starvation diet, and the lives of many of those with Type 1 diabetes ended in a diabetic coma and death. At first, the only available source of insulin was derived from pigs and cows. However, in the late 1950s, as a result of the discovery of the structure of insulin, it became possible to synthesise human insulin in the laboratory. Today, there is a whole range of long-, medium- and short-acting types of insulin that allow people with diabetes who need to inject insulin to control their condition extremely effectively.

While the advent of insulin brought better diabetes control, doctors faced a new set of problems with the discovery that diabetes could cause the development of complications such as blindness and kidney disease. The further step forward in treatment began after 1946, when doctors began to realise that good control of diabetes could reduce this risk. From the 1990s to the present, there has been an emphasis on controlling blood glucose levels, and more recently on controlling blood pressure and cholesterol levels, in an effort to avoid diabetic complications developing.

The role of diet

Diet has long been a cornerstone of diabetes management. For a long time – even after the era of the starvation diet – people with diabetes were advised to give up sweets, chocolates, cakes and pastries and weigh and measure all food carefully. Not surprisingly, the majority did not stick to this strict regimen. Foods labelled 'suitable for diabetics' are not recommended and are unnecessary. Today, the diet you will be recommended if you have diabetes is very similar to that suggested for the general population: a diet low in fat (especially saturated), salt and sugar; high in fibre; moderate amounts of protein; five portions of fruit and vegetables per day; limited alcohol; and with meals based around starchy foods. People with diabetes should also seek specialist advice and education from a state registered dietitian.

Current diabetes treatments

The aim of diabetes treatment for both Type 1 and Type 2 is to control blood glucose and blood pressure to minimise the risk of complications such as damage to the eyes, kidneys, nerves, heart and blood vessels. The exact treatments you are given will depend on the type of diabetes you have and how it affects you.

- **Type 1** is always treated by insulin injections, diet, exercise and lifestyle education.
- **Type 2** may be treated by diet and exercise alone, or by diet, exercise and medication. Around half of all people with Type 2 diabetes are prescribed medication. It's recently been recognised that Type 2 is a progressive condition, and if diet, exercise and tablets fail to control the condition, insulin may be needed.

Medications

Medications may include:

- **sulphonylureas (e.g. gliclazide, gilbenclamide):** which stimulate the pancreas to produce more insulin
- **biguanides (e.g. metformin):** which increases the effectiveness of available insulin
- **alpha-glucosidase inhibitor (e.g. acarbose):** which slows down the digestion of carbohydrates in order to prevent glucose being released so quickly into the bloodstream

- **prandial glucose regulators (e.g. repaglinide, nateglinide):** which stimulate the release of insulin in response to the body's blood glucose levels.
- **thiazolidinediones/'glitazones' (e.g. rosiglitazone, pioglitazone):** which help the body's insulin work more effectively

Testing the blood glucose

An important aspect of diabetes management is monitoring blood glucose levels. This helps the person with diabetes determine if their blood glucose level is within normal limits. If it is too low, which is known as hypoglycaemia, they will need to have a sugary drink followed by some form of long-acting carbohydrate; for example, a sandwich. If it is too high over a long period of time, their health care professional may suggest adjusting their dose of insulin or medication.

Preventive medications

However you are treated, the doctor may prescribe other, preventive medications such as blood pressure-lowering (anti-hypertensive) drugs and cholesterol-lowering drugs (e.g. statins) to protect against the development of possible complications.

Care patterns

Recently, efforts have gone into building a network of diabetes teams throughout the country to care for and support people with diabetes. At the heart of this is a multi-disciplinary team that will usually include your GP, a hospital consultant, specialist diabetes nurses and other health care professionals such as a podiatrist, ophthalmologist and dietitian (see Cavan, p.127). Community nurses, practice nurses and sometimes specialist diabetes nurses may visit you at home if you are older and housebound or have eyesight or other problems that would make it difficult for you to get to a clinic.

How does that measure up to treatment in the rest of Europe and the USA?

Although treatments are the same, in most of Europe diabetes care tends to be practised by specialist physicians rather than, as here, by a combination of GP and specialist care. In Scandinavia, where the health care system is similar to ours, people are cared for in the community and are sent to specialist diabetes centres for more complicated cases. Some devices, for instance insulin pumps, are more widely available in certain European countries such as Germany.

Treatments are broadly the same in the USA. New drug treatments, such as glitazones (see below), were first launched in the USA, and there is also a new combination therapy of a sulphonylurea combined with metformin for the treatment of Type 2 diabetes. New aids to diabetes control, such as the various blood glucose meters, often come on to the market sooner in the USA, and insulin pumps for the delivery of insulin are more widely used. However, diabetes care is very different from that in the UK, with most people seeing office-based diabetologists and a number of separate specialists for any complications that may occur. There is also a network of private diabetes educators and a small number of primary health care doctors, who operate rather like a mini-NHS system.

What new treatments are available?

A whole new class of diabetes drugs called thiazolidinediones, commonly known as glitazones, have come on to the market in the last few years, designed to treat insulin resistance. There is also a drug called nateglinide (Starlix), which is taken before meals to help modulate glucose levels. The use of a pump rather than injections to deliver insulin is another new development. A number of new blood glucose meters, which could cut the number of blood tests needed, are also becoming available. A host of new insulins, both short- and long-acting, are already available in the UK, and are designed to mimic more closely how the body itself produces insulin.

Can I get these on the NHS?

Glitazones, such as Rosiglitazone and Pioglitazone, are now available on the NHS, and more will emerge as new drugs receive approval. The National Institute for Clinical Excellence (NICE) is currently looking at the medical effectiveness and cost-effectiveness of insulin pumps, and is due to report early in 2003. NICE is also looking at insulin glargine (see p.116), a type of long-acting insulin.

What treatments are in the pipeline?

- **New formulations of current diabetes drugs:** for example a once-daily metformin should be available soon.

- **New insulins:** a number of short- and long-acting insulins tailored to meet individual needs, are being developed. The first of these (indeed the first new type of insulin for 60 years), insulin glargine, has recently been launched in the UK. It is a long-acting insulin that works slowly over 24 hours, and may have to be combined with another type of shorter-acting insulin or with diabetes medication to control blood glucose.
- **Needle-free insulin delivery systems:** inhaled insulin, in which a powder cloud of insulin is delivered into the lungs using a special inhaler, insulin mouth sprays (buccal insulin) and a system that forces a fine stream of insulin through a special nozzle, enabling insulin to penetrate the skin without the need for injection, are currently under research trials.
- **Drugs to treat eye problems:** research is also being conducted into new drugs to prevent visual problems caused by diabetes. These include a class of drugs called protein kinase C inhibitors (PKC), which slow the progression of diabetic retinopathy.
- **Less invasive (needle-free) blood glucose meters:** scientists are also evaluating new ways of monitoring blood sugar; for example, a new monitor using infrared sensors capable of reading glucose levels is currently being developed.
- **Research:** currently pancreatic cell transplants are being piloted, and stem cell therapy, designed to replace the failing pancreas, is also being researched.
- **An initiative called Dose Adjustment for Normal Eating (DAFNE):** this is under way in the UK designed to give patients with diabetes much more freedom to eat as they choose. This educational programme teaches people to adjust their insulin doses and then look at what they are cooking and eating, and calculate how much insulin they need to take for themselves (Humphriss, p.129).

Who treats it?

A GP, diabetes specialist nurse, endocrinologist and/or diabetologist, although according to Diabetes UK, approximately one in five strategic health authorities in the UK have the recommended number of consultants per head of the population.

What training will the specialist have?

Before becoming a consultant, your doctor will have had a general medical training, which includes five years at university followed by one year as a House Officer, before gaining registration with the General Medical Council. They will then have spent two to three years as a Senior House Officer in various medical disciplines. This will have been followed by a five- or six-year period of specialist registrar training, working in different hospitals specialising in diabetes, leading to a Certificate of Completion of Specialist Training that is recognised throughout Europe. In the fifth year and after their certification, doctors are encouraged to train to become sub-specialists.

Where will I receive care?

Provided your diabetes is well controlled, most of your basic care can be carried out by your GP at a GP-led diabetes clinic. Some GPs also run mini-clinics in partnership with consultants from the local hospital. You may be seen at a diabetes outpatient clinic based in your local hospital, or sometimes you may be referred to a specialist diabetes centre at a larger hospital (see Barnett, p.124). You may need to see your diabetes care team if:

- your diabetes is difficult to control
- you need to start treating your diabetes with insulin, having previously been treated with medication
- you are developing foot problems
- you have a high risk of developing heart problems; for example, if you have raised blood pressure and/or high levels of blood fats
- you have developed kidney problems
- you are a young person with Type 1 diabetes
- insulin dosage needs to be adjusted to achieve better control
- you are pregnant
- you need to be screened for eyesight problems if this is not done elsewhere
- you are a child with diabetes.

What questions should I ask about my treatment?

- Who will be in charge of my treatment?
- How often will I have to visit the diabetes clinic?

- Will I be treated with drugs or with insulin?
- What drugs will be prescribed and how do they act?
- How often will I have to take them?
- What side-effects can I expect?
- If I experience side-effects, are there any alternatives that can be prescribed?
- How do I monitor my blood glucose levels?
- How many times a day and when do I need to do this?
- Will I need to change my diet?
- Will I have to stop eating sugary foods?
- Are there any special precautions I need to take before exercise?
- How often should I exercise and what type of exercise should I do?
- If I am prescribed insulin, what type of insulin will it be?
- How often will I have to inject?
- What should I do to prevent hypoglycaemia?
- If I do experience hypoglycaemia, what should I do?
- Will I need to take blood pressure-lowering drugs?
- Will I need to take cholesterol-lowering drugs?
- Will I need to change my treatment if I plan to become pregnant?
- What about breastfeeding?
- How will my diabetes be managed if I have to go into hospital?

What will my treatment involve?

Initial management

When you are first diagnosed, you should receive a full medical examination and the diabetes multi-disciplinary team will work with you to develop an individual programme of care. You should have the chance to talk about your individual treatment with the diabetes specialist nurse or practice nurse, who should show you how to inject insulin (if necessary), how to monitor your blood glucose and how to recognise and deal with hypoglycaemia. You should also talk to a state registered dietitian, who can discuss your diet and exercise regime and help you make any adjustments that are necessary.

Continued care

Once your diabetes has been brought under reasonable control, you should have an annual appointment with a doctor skilled and experienced in diabetes. This could be either in general practice or at the hospital, depending on whether your GP takes an active role in the management of diabetes. You should have access to your diabetes care team to talk about how diabetes is affecting your everyday life and to discuss any issues or problems such as smoking, drinking alcohol, stress, sexual problems, physical activity, diet and weight control. The clinic should also encourage you to bring your partner, relatives or friends to support you, or your carer, so they can be kept informed about your diabetes management. At your annual review the following checks should be performed:

- blood testing to measure your long-term blood glucose control
- urine and blood tests to check for protein, an indication of kidney function
- blood tests to measure levels of blood fats
- a physical examination, including weight and blood pressure, with checks on your legs and feet to spot circulatory problems and your eyes to make sure you're not developing diabetic retinopathy.

What makes a REAL difference to controlling diabetes?

Until recently, diabetes care has been something of a postcode lottery. However, with the introduction of the Government's National Service Framework, diabetes services should be more standardised and evenly distributed throughout the country.

- **Access to a multi-disciplinary team.** They will work with you to control your diabetes as well as possible.
- **Self-management.** Ultimately, you have to live with your diabetes. Knowing how to manage your condition for yourself in everyday life is absolutely crucial to good diabetic control.
- **Structured care.** It should be organised so that you are recalled for an annual review (see above).
- **Integrated heart disease risk management.** Several large-scale studies have shown that treatment of high blood pressure and high blood cholesterol can save lives.

What is the difference between a well-run and a badly run diabetes service?

Continuity of care

Ideally you should see the same team of doctors and nurses each time you visit the clinic. Unfortunately, even with the best will in the world this is not always possible. However, there should be structures and procedures in place to make sure that the team knows your medical history and the course of your condition.

Accessibility

You should be able to contact any member of your diabetes team for advice whenever you need it, either by visiting the clinic or by phone.

Education

A well-run diabetes service will provide ongoing education to make sure you properly understand diabetes and how it affects you. It should also provide special tutorial sessions on any issues affecting you; for example, diet and weight management, exercise or foot care.

Partnership

A well-run service should recognise you as a member of the diabetes management team and encourage you to take an active part in your treatment and care (see Cavan, p.126).

Will I get better treatment if I go privately?

Almost certainly not. There is very little private diabetes care in this country, as the insurance companies don't provide cover for chronic, long-term illnesses such as diabetes. Also, if you go private you will not have the advantage of being cared for by a multi-disciplinary team (see Cavan, p.127) .

Will I get better treatment if I go abroad?

On the whole, no. Although there is a shortage of specialists in the UK, the development of multi-disciplinary teams and specialised diabetes services means that treatment in this country is improving. Because diabetes is a chronic condition that needs regular monitoring, you are better off using a local service where you can get consistent advice and care.

What support will I be offered by the clinic, and are there any independent support groups I can join?

The clinic should make sure you have a full range of up-to-date written and other information on any aspect of diabetes that may affect you. They should give you back-up and help with any measures you may need to take, such as informing the DVLA if you are a driver, and give you details about services provided by Diabetes UK and any local diabetes groups. The team should also be easy to contact if you have any worries about your treatment.

Useful addresses

Diabetes Insight
www.diabetes-insight.org
An information website and online support forum for people
with diabetes.

Diabetes UK
10 Parkway
London NW1 7AA
Tel 020 7424 1000
Careline 020 7424 1030 (voice) (9 am to 5 pm Monday to Friday)
020 7424 1888 (text) (9 am to 5 pm Monday to Friday)
Email: info@diabetes.org.uk
Email: careline@diabetes.org.uk
www.diabetes.org.uk

International Diabetes Federation
Avenue Emile De Mot 19
B-1000 Brussels
Belgium
Tel +322 5385511

Juvenile Diabetes Research Foundation
19 Angel Gate
City Road
London EC1V 2PT
Tel 020 7713 2030
www.jdrf.org.uk

Expert opinions

Professor Anthony Barnett

The UK is facing a diabetes epidemic that can only be managed by increased emphasis on public health and education, and a fundamental reorganisation of services, says Professor Tony Barnett, head of one of the largest diabetes units in the country at Birmingham Heartlands Hospital.

'If you look at the epidemiological projection, the suggestion is that by the year 2025, with the present rate of increase in the condition, we are going to be spending one quarter of the total healthcare budget of the UK on diabetes and its complications,' he says. 'We are already spending 10 per cent, and in the States they are spending 15 per cent. These are massive figures.'

Our increasingly unhealthy lifestyles are at the heart of the problem. Obesity and inactivity, together with the fact that we are living longer, mean that the current 1.4 million diabetes sufferers will have swelled to 3 million by 2010. And it is not just adults who are at risk. The increase in Type 2 diabetes among children is particularly worrying, as just a few years ago this form of the disease was virtually unheard of in people under the age of 40. 'We are now seeing Type 2 diabetes in teenage children,' says Barnett. 'Where there is a high ethnic population, there are now almost as many kids with Type 2 diabetes as there are with Type 1, which is the traditional young-onset type of diabetes.'

The costs of treating diabetes alone would be high, but people with diabetes are also at increased risk of a host of other conditions, draining healthcare resources further. 'Diabetes is the commonest cause of blindness in the working population in the UK. It is also the single commonest cause of kidney disease that needs dialysis. But crucially, it is also an extremely important risk factor for heart disease,' he says. 'About 80 per cent of patients with diabetes die from cardiovascular disease, many of them prematurely.'

There is no clear consensus yet on how to curb the alarming rise in diabetes prevalence, and Barnett feels that there is still insufficient interest at the highest level for the sort of major initiatives that would be needed. 'If you think about the vast amount the fast food industry spends on advertising, compared to the minuscule amount the Government spends on public health issues, you know we're losing. The Government is going to have to be prepared to say that they are going to put a lot of resources in, just like they've done with cigarette smoking and AIDS. And I don't see the appetite for that with any of the Government representatives that I've dealt with.'

Another possibility would be to actively screen for people who are likely to become diabetic, as treatment of this group, who are described as 'glucose intolerant', has been shown to delay the onset of diabetes. But again, there are problems of scale, as even a selective screening programme, covering risk groups such as ethnic minorities, people with high blood pressure or the over-50s, would probably end up including almost 50 per cent of the adult population and be extremely expensive.

In the absence of effective preventive measures, existing diabetes services are going to have to adapt to the increasing number of patients, and Barnett feels that a major reorganisation is needed. 'We're talking potentially of about three million people, and there are just not enough specialists to cope with those kinds of numbers,' he says. 'GPs are going to have to become more involved, but there are now quite a lot of GPs who are actually very interested in diabetes and are willing to take on more and more of the load.'

In addition to the shift in diabetes care from hospital specialists to GPs, improvements will be needed at the interface between the two. At the Birmingham unit, a number of initiatives to achieve this are already being explored. GPs come to the unit and work alongside its specialist staff, and a consultant-level doctor is going to be appointed to work away from the unit in the community. Barnett hopes that these changes will reduce the unit's routine workload, while helping to identify more quickly those in need of specialist care.

The unit itself has facilities to ensure that patients see an appropriate specialist quickly, which is important in tackling the many risks associated with diabetes. 'We have a general clinic, where things like annual reviews can be done, which is basically the diabetic patient's equivalent of an MOT, but we also have a special clinic for every complication,' he says. 'For example, if someone develops diabetic kidney disease, they will see a diabetes specialist and a kidney specialist in the same room at a joint clinic that is held every week.'

Similar dedicated clinics are held for obesity, adolescents and children, foot problems, eye complications, erectile dysfunction and more. But this range of services is far from universal among UK diabetes units, and Barnett thinks that this is an area where patients should push for change or look elsewhere. 'At least 50 per cent of diabetes services do not provide those kind of facilities,' he says. 'Patients need to ask themselves if the service they are attending is providing for their requirements. When they come to the clinic, are they being fobbed off by people saying, "Yes, we would like you to see the kidney specialist but actually there is a six-month wait for that."'

Delays in seeing a specialist can lead to unnecessary complications, so denying patients these clinics is a false economy. For example, at King's College Hospital in London, the introduction of a foot-care service held jointly with chiropodists, expert shoe-fitters and vascular surgeons, reduced the amputation rate by two-thirds. This kind of improvement will be needed across the board if UK diabetes services are to cope with the projected increase in people developing the disease.

Dr David Cavan

Some UK diabetes services are failing to address the educational and psychological needs of their patients, according to Dr David Cavan, a consultant diabetologist at the Bournemouth Diabetes and Endocrine Centre, which is part of the Royal Bournemouth Hospital. 'There is still too much of a legacy in diabetes care that if the diabetes is badly controlled it's the patient's fault,' he says. 'It is a very paternalistic attitude that can come through, which fails to recognise the many factors that can lead to poor control and the difficult task patients face in achieving good control of their diabetes.'

Diabetes is a long-term condition that affects every body system, and while patients are monitored and advised by their GPs or a hospital specialist service from time to time, day-to-day control of the condition is in the patient's hands. Poor control of blood sugar levels contributes to serious problems further down the line, an effect that can be seen in the significant numbers of diabetic patients who go on to suffer from heart disease, strokes, kidney failure and other complications.

'If you can provide people with the tools to look after themselves early on, then you can prevent an awful lot of problems,' says Cavan. 'If I was looking for a good diabetes service, I would want evidence that there is real patient involvement and education from very early on. In our centre, for example, all newly diagnosed patients attend a structured education and management programme, which we have shown leads to good diabetic control, sustained over several years.'

This education can be as simple as explaining what each treatment offered is actually for, as people often fail to take medicines that do not appear to have an immediate effect. 'If you are going to put a patient on a tablet, they need to know why they are going on that tablet. Many of the conditions associated with diabetes (such as high levels of blood sugar, cholesterol or blood pressure) are asymptomatic. We prescribe tablets, but unless there's a clear understanding of why they're needed patients may not take them because the treatment doesn't make them feel any better. Patients need to know that if they take these tablets and get their blood pressure and cholesterol down, they are going to protect their hearts and brains in the future.'

While the consultant diabetologist has a role to play in patient education, the overall standard of care is highly dependent on the whole team, which will also include specialist nurses and dietitians. For this reason, Cavan feels that patients are not necessarily well advised to look to the private sector for diabetes care. 'In other areas of medicine such as surgery, for example, your main focus will be on the person doing the operation. Diabetes is long term and affects most areas of daily life, and so you need a team approach. For this reason, diabetes care in the private sector may be more fragmented, because you may not have the rest of the team (nurse or dietitian, for example) readily available.'

Even a well-designed diabetes service can only help patients to manage their disease if they are motivated to do so, and Cavan is studying the mental health of diabetes sufferers in the hope of addressing this. 'There is plenty of evidence that up to 40 per cent of people with diabetes have some sort of mental health problem. At its mildest it could just be a degree of anxiety about their diabetes, but depression is very common, and generally this is completely ignored.'

'People who are suffering from these problems can get an awful lot of advice and input from specialists and nurses and dietitians, but at the end of the day they are only going to get their diabetes under control if they are sufficiently motivated themselves.' The Bournemouth unit is currently testing the effectiveness of integrated psychological counselling in diabetes management, and Cavan hopes that this approach will help to tackle this widespread problem in the future.

Another area under investigation is the use of IT systems to optimise the insulin doses of patients with Type 1 diabetes. Patients are asked to collect data on their blood sugar levels, insulin doses and food intake for a few days. Using a sophisticated computer model, the data are used to predict what their ideal insulin dose should be. At present, the system is used as part of a patient education programme, but a pilot project is under way whereby patients use the system via the internet to optimise their treatment themselves. 'The vision is that if you have got a problem with diabetic control, rather than being dependent on someone else to sort it out, you can collect some data, enter it into your computer and get feedback whenever you want.'

This project represents another step towards increased patient empowerment in diabetes care, and this is the direction that holds the most promise for the future, in Cavan's view. However, for patients to take charge of managing their disease, they must have access to comprehensive education services, and their mental health needs must also be addressed.

Dr David Humphriss

An education programme that has been significantly improving the quality of life for patients with Type 1 diabetes in Germany for around 15 years is now beginning to filter through to UK diabetes patients, says Dr David Humphriss, who runs one of the centres where the initiative is being tried. The programme, called Dose Adjustment for Normal Eating (DAFNE), is designed to give patients with diabetes much more freedom to eat as they choose.

'Essentially, it is a five-day educational course for patients with Type 1 diabetes, and it covers pretty much every educational topic they need to know about. Specifically, it teaches patients to count the amount of carbohydrate in their meals and then calculate how much insulin they should take to balance that carbohydrate up,' says Humphriss.

In the past, doctors calculated the insulin dose, then patients had to work out their meals to match the amount. 'The concept has now been turned on its head,' says Humphriss. 'The doctor shouldn't be deciding how much you eat – you should be deciding whether you are hungry or not.'

DAFNE teaches people to adjust their background insulin doses and then look at what they are cooking and eating, and calculate how much short-acting insulin they need to take for themselves. In addition to greater empowerment for patients, the approach delivers significant clinical benefits. 'In Germany, they have been seeing an improvement in blood sugar control, but they also have been seeing a massive increase in quality of life scores. The patients are happier – they turn up at hospital less and they turn up at work more.'

Humphriss runs the diabetes service at Scarborough General Hospital, one of ten centres nationally where DAFNE is being tested. Initial trials sponsored by Diabetes UK in three other centres in the UK indicate that it will offer similar benefits to UK patients. It is currently undergoing appraisal by the National Institute for Clinical Excellence and, if approved, it could be rolled out nationally.

Scarborough was selected to participate in the DAFNE trial because it is a typical small, rural diabetes service, facing a very different set of problems to the larger urban units. 'The advantage of the bigger centres is in numbers of staff. Yes, they have more patients to look after, but by simple numbers of staff, they have people who can take a specialist interest in particular areas of diabetes: kidneys and diabetes, cardiology and diabetes, feet and diabetes, whatever,' says Humphriss. 'We're really not in a position to do that. There are two consultants, a staff grade and a specialist registrar. When you add together all the specialist nurses, podiatrists, dietitians and administrative staff, there are fewer than 20 of us in total.'

Inevitably, stretching limited resources over a wide area results in some compromises, and smaller services cannot offer as great a range of joint clinics for diabetes-related complications as the larger centres. However, the system at Scarborough does still provide fairly rapid access to the different specialists. 'Our local renal physicians are based 50 miles away, and they are here one day a week. They are incredibly busy, and there is no way we could do a joint clinic. But they see our patients when they are in town and provide an excellent service – that is the way rural medicine works.'

Humphriss feels that smaller services also have benefits for patients in terms of a less intimidating environment and a greater opportunity to get to know the staff. 'At a large service, there can be 100 or 150 patients cramming in to the outpatient department for the afternoon, and that is not a terribly pleasant experience. The smaller service, where there are maybe two doctors, a dietitian, a specialist nurse and a podiatrist, is a much more pleasant experience for them. They are much more likely to see the same people every time, which gives them continuity.'

At the end of the day, both large and small diabetes services have benefits and drawbacks, and both will be needed to manage the ever-increasing numbers of UK diabetes patients. Although resources are limited, Humphriss believes that initiatives like DAFNE that seek to improve the service delivered and tailor it to the needs of patients can offer cost-effective solutions to some of the problems facing patients at the moment.

Heart disease

What is the specialty?
Cardiology and cardiac surgery.

What is heart disease?
The term 'heart disease' covers a number of conditions, including problems with the heart muscle, the valves, the rhythm of the heart (arrhythmias) and congenital heart disease, which is when you are born with an abnormality in the structure of the heart. By far the most common type of heart disease is ischaemic heart disease, or coronary artery disease, which develops when the coronary artery becomes narrowed by a build-up of fatty material called atheroma and the blood supply to the heart is insufficient. This section uses the term 'heart disease' to mean coronary artery disease, which is one of the biggest health problems in the UK. Coronary artery disease usually leads to a heart attack if left untreated. Its symptoms include:

- **Angina:** a feeling of heaviness or tightness in the centre of the chest, which can spread to the arms, neck, back or stomach and which can last for a few seconds or minutes. The tightness can be severe in some people, whereas for others it is not much more than mild discomfort.
- **Ischaemia:** a lack of blood to the heart, which may not have any warning signs.
- **Thrombosis:** the formation of a blood clot, which blocks the flow of blood through an artery. When a blood clot develops in a coronary artery it is called a coronary thrombosis and is very likely to lead to a heart attack.

Drugs and lifestyle changes can help control angina attacks and the build-up of atheroma in the blood vessels, but they cannot reverse damage that has already been done to the heart – they can only help stop it getting any worse.

The risk of developing coronary heart disease is increased by a number of lifestyle factors, including being overweight, a lack of regular exercise, smoking, poor diet, excessive alcohol consumption, high cholesterol level and high blood pressure. However, these risk factors do not explain all cases of coronary heart disease, and research is also under way into non-conventional factors such as the role of infection (see Kaski, p.146).

What are the statistics?

In the UK more people die from coronary artery disease than from any other disease. According to the British Heart Foundation, just under 45,000 people died from the disease in 2000 and around 270,000 people have heart attacks each year in the UK. The death rate from coronary heart disease in the UK is among the highest in the world. Among developed countries, only Ireland and Finland have a higher rate than the UK. Death rates are higher in Scotland, Northern Ireland and the north of England than in Wales and the south of England.

How is it currently treated?

Since 1938, when an Amercian surgeon, Robert Gross, performed the first heart surgery, drugs and techniques for treating heart disease have evolved dramatically. The treatment you will be offered will depend on the degree of angina or the likelihood of you having a heart attack.

Medications

The majority of patients with coronary heart disease are treated with drugs rather than surgery. There are several classes of drugs that have effects on the heart and/or arteries, and treatment depends on your specific problems. Some drugs have more than one effect, and for the conditions listed below you may be given any of the drugs mentioned:

- **High cholesterol levels:** treated with cholesterol-lowering drugs, mainly from a class of drugs called statins.
- **Blood pressure:** can be lowered with a variety of drugs, e.g. ACE inhibitors, diuretics, beta-blockers and calcium-channel blockers.
- **Angina:** nitrates help relieve the pain of this condition.
- **Heart failure:** the effects can be improved by diuretics, which are often combined with digoxin or ACE inhibitors.
- **Heart arrhythmia:** anti-arrhythmic drugs can correct heart rhythm, and anticoagulants (e.g. heparin or warfarin) are used to prevent blood clots forming in patients who are unable to take aspirin.
- **Valvular heart disease:** the symptoms can be treated with ACE inhibitors, digoxin and diuretics.
- **Blood clots:** aspirin helps prevent these forming.

Surgery

If you are taking the medication you have been prescribed and have made any necessary lifestyle changes, but your symptoms are getting worse, you may be given a cardiac catheterisation test to find out where your arteries are narrowed and how narrow they are. Coronary angiography is the gold standard catheterisation test, but it carries a small risk of serious complications and requires skill to perform. The Government has suggested that hospitals that do this test should perform at least 500 per year (see Shapiro, p.148). You can search the Dr Foster website to see if your hospital meets this target.

If the tests shows that one or more of your arteries has severe narrowing or a blockage, your chances of having a heart attack in the near future are high and you may be advised to have revascularisation therapy, which is where the blocked blood vessels are widened or replaced with grafts. Revascularisation treatments include:

- **Coronary angioplasty.** The walls of the narrow arteries are stretched, which helps break up the fatty deposit and allows the blood to flow more freely. The technique has developed rapidly since it was first used in 1977 and is now a common treatment for coronary artery disease. Over 20,000 angioplasties are done each year in the UK. Angioplasty avoids the need for a major operation. However, people who have angioplasty are more likely to get angina again than people who have bypass surgery, so they may be more likely to need further treatment or heart surgery later. Angioplasty is a very specialised technique and requires great skill and experience.

- **Coronary artery bypass graft.** Sections of blood vessels are removed from other parts of the body and grafted on to the aorta to bypass the damaged coronary arteries and give the blood another route to the heart. In just a few decades this technique has gone from being a new, experimental treatment to being a relatively safe, routine procedure that can add decades to people's lives. Bypass surgery has a more long-term result than angioplasty but is a major operation and is reserved for more life-threatening cases. You can check the Dr Foster website (www.drfoster.co.uk) for the mortality rates for each hospital performing this operation and what percentage of patients are operated on within six months of referral (see Angelini, p.142).

If you do suffer a heart attack, your chances of surviving depend on how quickly you get to hospital and how soon you are treated. Thrombolysis, which involves giving clot-busting drugs, is the standard treatment in the UK for heart attacks, but its effectiveness depends on it being done quickly. Hospitals aim to perform thrombolysis within 30 minutes of a heart-attack patient entering the hospital, but many hospitals don't reach this target. You can check the Dr Foster website for a list of those hospitals that do currently.

How does that measure up to treatment in the rest of Europe and the USA?

In many European countries, particularly France and Germany, cardiology services are very well developed, with many more specialist facilities than in the UK, and surgical procedures to treat coronary artery disease are more widely available. The main reason for this is the lack of funds in the NHS, although a shortage of medical personnel contributes to the comparatively low number of operations carried out here. The UK has about one-thirtieth of the number of specialist cardiologists there are in the USA. Germany has ten times as many consultants as the UK. However, USA cardiologists are far less specialised than cardiologists in the UK.

Another difference is that in some US hospitals they use angioplasty to treat heart attacks (known as primary angioplasty). There is a lot of evidence that primary angioplasty is the best treatment for a heart attack, but it is not a routine treatment option in the UK.

What new treatments are available?

Drug therapy for cardiology stabilised about five years ago and there have been few new medications in recent years. Surgically, each technique is constantly being refined and new tools and methods evaluated. One exciting new development is coating with a drug the stainless steel mesh, known as a stent, which helps support the arteries after angioplasty. The pharmacological coating is believed to reduce the blockage of the artery after angioplasty.

Can I get these on the NHS?

All classes of drugs used to treat heart disease are widely available under the NHS. The new, coated stent is currently being trialled at the Royal Brompton Hospital and looks likely to become the gold standard treatment available on the NHS.

What treatments are in the pipeline?

One exciting new area of research, which is at animal experimental stage, is in using hormone growth factor to regrow arteries. Instead of having to carry out a bypass operation to treat coronary artery disease, doctors inject growth factors to develop new branches of arteries. Another important area is in understanding the link between cardiovascular disease and hormone replacement therapy (see Kaski, p.145). There have also been developments in terms of identifying patients at risk using chemical markers, rather than just high cholesterol levels and high blood pressure. Research by the leading doctors we profile here is already leading to improvements in clinical practice: initiatives like the heart valve registry (Taylor, p.151); research into the mechanisms that cause arteries to narrow (Kaski, p.145); the pioneering work into mechanical heart pumps (Westaby, p.152–4) and the techniques being developed for correcting heart disease without the need for open heart surgery (Shapiro, p.148).

Who treats it?

If your GP suspects you have heart disease, you will be referred to a heart specialist (cardiologist) for tests and any necessary treatment, including surgery. Your cardiologist will send results of the tests and details of any treatment you need to your GP. He or she will coordinate your care, give you advice and information, carry out or organise any regular tests you require, and may prescribe your medication.

What training will the specialist have?

Before becoming a consultant, your doctor will have had a general medical training, which includes five years at university followed by one year as a House Officer, before gaining registration with the General Medical Council. They will then have spent two to three years as a Senior House Officer in various medical disciplines. This is followed by a five- or six-year period of specialist registrar training in cardiology, working in different hospitals, leading to a Certificate of

Completion of Specialist Training that is recognised throughout Europe. In the fifth year and post-certification, doctors are encouraged to train to become sub-specialists.

Where will I receive care?

You will see your cardiologist at the outpatient department at the hospital or clinic from which they work. If you are admitted to hospital in an emergency, you will see your consultant on the ward. However, remember that your consultant is only one member of a team, and if you require surgery, there is no certainty that he or she will perform your operation. Your surgeon will always meet you before the operation.

What questions should I ask about my treatment?

It is important you are fully informed about any procedure that you are to undergo, the experience of the consultant conducting the operation and the results of the unit in that particular procedure. Your consultant should be able to answer all relevant questions, which may include the following:

- Who is going to carry out the operation?
- How many times has the surgeon carried out this procedure?
- What is the mortality rate of the surgeon?
- What is the rate of complications for the surgeon?
- How many of these operations do you do as a unit?
- What is the mortality rate of the unit?
- What is the rate of complications for the unit?
- What are the benefits of the operation compared with not having it done?
- What are the risks involved and what can be done to minimise these?
- Are there any alternatives to surgery?
- How long is the expected recovery time?

What will my treatment involve?

Angioplasty involves inserting a fine, hollow tube called a catheter, with a small inflatable balloon at its tip, into an artery in your groin or arm under local anaesthetic. The surgeon uses X-ray screening to show the blood vessels and to help them direct the catheter to a coronary artery. When the catheter reaches a narrowed section the balloon is inflated so that it flattens the deposits in the artery, which should start to break up. Another set of X-rays is then taken to make sure that the blood flow has improved. If it hasn't, the procedure is repeated before the catheter is removed. The catheter usually contains a stainless-steel mesh, called a stent, which holds open the artery walls. After the balloon is deflated and removed, the stent is left in place to give support to the artery walls and help to stop them narrowing again. You can expect to stay in hospital for one to two days and you can usually return to work after about a week.

After angioplasty, the arteries may get narrow again in time. However, the use of stents has greatly reduced the risk of this happening. According to the British Heart Foundation, around nine out of every ten angioplasties are successful. The risks include heart attack, stroke or dying: about five people in every thousand (0.5 per cent) die within 30 days of having the operation.

A coronary artery bypass graft (CABG) may be a better option than angioplasty if your coronary arteries are very narrow and/or contain large deposits. The aim of this technique is to bypass the narrowed sections of coronary arteries. You may be offered a bypass if you have had unsuccessful angioplasty or if there is a high chance you will have a heart attack in the near future.

A bypass is a major operation involving a general anaesthetic. A long cut is made down the chest and through the breastbone. The heart is stopped during the operation and a heart–lung machine is used to provide blood and oxygen to the body's organs (see Taylor, p.151, for work on improvements to the design of these machines). Professor Gianni Angelini, profiled on p.142, has played an important role in popularising beating heart bypass surgery, in which, rather than stopping the heart completely, only a small area is immobilised to allow the surgeon to operate. The surgeon will detach an artery from your chest wall and sew or graft its open end onto the damaged coronary artery just below the blockage. Another option is to take a length of vein from your leg and graft one end to your aorta and the other to the coronary artery below the blockage. Whichever method is used, the blood will then be able to flow to your heart through the grafted blood vessel, bypassing the damaged coronary artery.

After the operation you will be looked after in either an intensive therapy unit (ITU), an intensive care unit (ICU), a cardiac recovery unit or a coronary care unit (CCU). These units have the sophisticated medical equipment needed to monitor your progress for the first 24 to 48 hours after your operation. When your condition is stable you'll be taken to a cardiac surgical ward or a high dependency unit. You can expect to stay in hospital for seven to ten days. Before you are discharged you will be given enough medication to last you for a few days and a letter for your GP with details about the drugs you need (which your GP will prescribe for you) and any other information about your treatment. You will need to have two to three months off work and it can take up to six months before you feel normal.

Over 28,000 patients have coronary artery bypass surgery in the UK each year. The risk of dying within 30 days of a first operation is about three in every 100 patients. Between one and two in every 100 patients require bypass surgery again within six months, and around seven in every 100 within five years. However, around seven in every ten patients who have a bypass operation get immediate relief from angina, lasting for at least five years. The remainder find that the bypass improves their angina.

What makes a REAL difference to getting better?

The most important aspect to recovering from heart disease is cardiac rehabilitation, which involves structured training, advice and help in diet, stopping smoking and beginning to exercise. Other critical factors are being on the right drugs long-term and, if you require it, surgical intervention. If surgery is needed, then the outcomes of the surgeon as well as the outcomes and facilities of the unit are important (see Shapiro, p.148).

What is the difference between a well-run and a badly run clinic?

A good coronary care unit or intensive care unit should have modern, up-to-date equipment for monitoring patients after major surgery and for dealing with emergencies such as cardiac or respiratory arrest. The unit should be well laid out, with enough room for staff to use emergency equipment at the side of each bed and to be able to see all the patients in the unit. Intensive care is a specialised area of medicine, and a good coronary care unit will also have a resident doctor and nurses who are well trained and experienced in caring for seriously ill patients and treating the potential complications of major surgery. It is an added advantage if a consultant who is a specialist in coronary or intensive care is in charge of the unit.

Will I get better treatment if I go privately?

Almost all consultants who work in private hospitals also have NHS practices and therefore the quality of treatment is likely to be much the same, whether private or NHS. If you do choose to have surgery in a private hospital, it is important to find out what facilities they have should any complications arise. Not all private hospitals have the range of emergency equipment available at the larger NHS hospitals. However, on the plus side, if you do have private treatment, you will bypass NHS waiting lists and have the reassurance of knowing that your consultant will perform your operation. Nursing care is also theoretically better in private hospitals because there is a higher nurse–patient ratio.

Will I get better treatment if I go abroad?

Since July 2002, all patients who have been waiting more than six months for a heart operation have had the option to travel to Europe, where the treatment will remain free. Whether or not you will receive better treatment depends on the facilities of the unit and the experience of the surgeon and the team. In terms of outcomes for surgical procedures, the UK is at the same level as the USA for bypass and better than Europe.

What support will I be offered by the clinic and are there any independent support groups I can join?

A cardiac rehabilitation nurse will visit you on the ward to give you advice and information about any rehabilitation programmes or health support groups in your area. If you have had coronary bypass surgery, hospital staff will want to be sure that there will be someone at home to help look after you for the first couple of weeks. If there is no one who can stay with you, arrangements can be made for a district nurse and/or home help to visit you regularly for a few days. Although cardiac rehabilitation programmes have been shown to improve people's life expectancy after a heart attack or heart surgery, they are not run by all hospitals. If there isn't one at your hospital, ask your doctor for details of any that are available in your area.

The British Heart Foundation is a good independent source of information, advice and support. The Foundation employs seven cardiac support advisers, whose role is to promote and encourage patient support groups. Contact the British Heart Foundation for details of a support group in your area.

Useful addresses

British Cardiac Patients Association
Unit 5D, 2 Station Road
Swavesy
Cambridge CB4 5QJ
Tel 01954 202022

British Cardiac Society
9 Fitzroy Square
London W1T 5HW
Tel 020 7383 3887
www.bcs.com

British Heart Foundation
14 Fitzhardinge Street
London W1H 6DH
Tel 020 7935 0185
www.bhf.org.uk

Expert opinions

Professor Gianni Angelini

Professor Gianni Angelini is a leading heart surgeon and the head of the Bristol Heart Institute, a centre with an international reputation for innovation and research in heart surgery, together with one of the best patient survival rates in the country. He has led the move towards greater openness in surgery, and believes strongly in patients having access to information about the performance of individual units.

In heart surgery, key pieces of information include the unit's mortality rate, the volume of operations it performs and its rates for complications. This information is not universally available to the public at present. However, Bristol has taken a lead in this area by publishing all of its results on the internet since 1996, and Angelini believes that this openness has not only helped GPs and patients to find the right surgeon but has also improved standards at the unit as a whole. 'It suddenly focused everybody's minds on the job. Because we were collecting information, which we had made a commitment to publish and make available to the general public, there was a considerable incentive for everybody to double their efforts. As a consequence of this, we have good results.'

Even when results are not publicly available, Angelini believes that it is important for patients to discuss them with their surgeon during consultation. 'If I was a patient, I would say, "How many of these operations do you do as a unit? How many do you do personally? What is your mortality? And what is your rate of complication in terms of stroke or in terms of infection?" These are fairly straightforward questions, and they would be pretty easy to answer.'

Although all the surgeons at a unit will have their own results for the various procedures on offer, it is also important for prospective patients to find out about the centre as a whole. 'The surgeon, contrary to general belief, is only one member of the team. If we didn't have a first-class intensive care unit, we would never have had these results,' he adds.

The Bristol unit certainly has nothing to hide, as its results are significantly better than the UK average. Angelini believes that the centre's varied research interests contribute to its clinical success. 'When you have a very active academic unit, you can take problems, try to find solutions and then implement those solutions,' he says.

'When I arrived in Bristol in 1992, we were doing things that we would now regard as obsolete. For example, from 1992–96 we used cold saline with potassium to stop the heart during surgery. In 1996 we changed to warm blood – the patient's own blood with potassium added to stop the heart. Recently, we have audited some of our results and discovered that from 1996 onward we had a very dramatic reduction in the incidence of complications like a myo-cardial infarction during surgery. This coincided, very simply, with changing one step of the surgical procedure, and this was based effectively on scientific evidence. First, what we were doing before wasn't working so well, and second, we had found a way to do it better.'

While the heart can now be protected more effectively when it is stopped, the procedure still carries risks. Angelini and his team have played an important part in popularising beating heart bypass surgery, in which, rather than stopping the heart completely, only a small area is immobilised to allow the surgeon to operate. 'Our results show that the technique offers a lot of early benefits over the conventional method,' he reports. 'I would say that about 30 per cent of heart bypass operations worldwide are now done using the method, and this is growing all the time. We do about 60 per cent as a unit, and I myself do around 90 per cent. Once you have enough experience, you can do almost any coronary bypass operation using the technique.'

In both his own research and his attitude to openness, Angelini has shown a willingness to break from the pack. But then he has an unusual background for a heart surgeon. He grew up in a small village outside Siena in Tuscany, and first qualified as a mechanical engineer. 'I always wanted to do medicine,' he says, 'but there was not enough money, so I took a shorter degree instead.'

It was his ability on the athletics track that provided the break. The team for which he was running offered to help him fund a medical course – a commitment they honoured even when his running career was cut short by hepatitis, contracted when training in Russia.

His interest in heart surgery began at medical school, and he secured an internship with a top heart surgeon in Florence. 'The unit in Florence was, funnily enough, completely staffed with nurses who were British, Australian and American,' he says. 'They told me that Great Britain was the best place to train, so I got a letter of introduction from one of these nurses and off I went to visit the Brompton Hospital in London. It was gut feeling more than common sense.'

After a six-month intensive language course, he obtained his first junior post in London and later became a registrar at the University Hospital of Wales in Cardiff, where he undertook most of his training. 'From Wales, I went for one year to Rotterdam in Holland to study paediatric and transplantation surgery. From there, I went via Wales to Sheffield as a consultant senior lecturer. And three years later I was appointed to the British Heart Foundation as chair of cardiac surgery in Bristol.'

Angelini believes that openness and communication are the most important qualities in a good heart surgeon. 'If you can communicate with people, tell them honestly what's going on, they will never complain. This is my personal experience. It's when you try to hide things or not interact, people get suspicious and then you get into trouble.'

Professor Juan Carlos Kaski

Heart disease is the biggest killer in the UK, and some of its causes are not well understood. Well-known risk factors like smoking and obesity undoubtedly have a major role to play in causing the narrowed arteries and heart problems of many sufferers. But a significant minority do not conform to the standard profile. Professor Juan Carlos Kaski heads the Coronary Artery Disease Research Unit at St George's Hospital in London, where researchers are studying atypical forms of the disease and the risk factors that contribute to them.

'I have found that 30 per cent of patients undergoing cardiac catheterisation for the diagnosis of chest pain have normal arteries. In many of these cases, the mechanism appears to be a dysfunction of the micro-vessels – the tiny arteries inside the heart muscle itself,' he says.

This form of the condition, known as cardiac syndrome X, appears to be particularly common in post-menopausal women, leading researchers to suspect a link to hormone levels. Elucidating the precise nature of this link, and looking at the effects of treatments like hormone replacement therapy (HRT) on the risk of developing heart disease, are priorities for Kaski's team.

One of the problems in relation to HRT in women who have been diagnosed with typical angina has been that the methods used to study the effect appear to be influencing the results, despite the encouraging results of observational studies. Newer prospective studies, in which groups of women are followed up over many years, have cast doubt on the theory that HRT can help to avoid the development of further cardiac events. 'For many years, we based our decisions on observational studies, which suggested that hormone replacement therapy was quite effective in improving survival and reducing cardiac events. But prospective studies carried out on women with coronary artery disease are not supporting the results of the observational studies. So there is a move worldwide to develop studies in a larger number of patients to clarify the issue.'

The St George's group is also studying the mechanisms that cause arteries to narrow. In this area, inflammation of the artery wall has emerged as a key contributory factor. 'By different mechanisms, cholesterol, hypertension, smoking and ageing will all stimulate inflammatory pathways in the arterial wall. So inflammation is, at this point in time, thought to be one of the key components of arteriosclerosis [atherosclerosis].'

This new understanding led researchers to look at other causes of inflammation of the arteries as possible contributors to heart disease. 'The conventional risk factors are extremely important, but ultimately we realise that they do not explain all the incident cases of coronary heart disease,' says Kaski. 'In other words, there are patients in whom these risk factors are not so prevalent, but they still develop serious heart conditions.'

Infection is one of the non-conventional factors that Kaski's team has been looking at, and while it is unlikely that infection alone could cause arteriosclerosis, it seems to compound the effects of other risk factors. 'Infection alone would be very unlikely to start arteriosclerosis. What it does is stimulate or accelerate the process. Essentially, it would be easier for a chronic infection to cause or facilitate vascular damage if the person has a history of smoking, high cholesterol or hypertension.'

Evidence of infection is often found in the deposits, or plaques, that narrow the arteries of coronary artery disease sufferers, especially those who have suffered from gum, bowel or lung infections, in which bacteria may have accessed the blood stream. Kaski's group have found that in these patients, treatment with antibiotics is enough to produce a marked improvement in heart and blood vessel function. In the future, it may be possible to develop vaccines that would stop bacteria from gaining a foothold in the first place, and this could significantly slow the progression of the disease.

With his history of looking beyond the conventional causes of heart disease, Kaski feels that it is very important for cardiologists to look at each case on its merit and not just offer the standard 'off-the-shelf' treatments. For patients themselves, the best way to ensure a high standard of care is to find out about their condition and request a referral to a centre that specialises in its treatment. 'I have ordinary cardiology referrals from GPs in the area who do not necessarily know of my special interests,' he says. 'But I also have another group of patients, who have been referred from different regions because they are aware of the research we are doing here. The patients themselves search the internet and ask their GPs to refer them to us for specialist treatment. We are seeing more and more of this, and it is very useful.'

The area of heart disease covers a large number of different conditions, and for those whose illness does not conform to the standard pattern there can be great benefits in being referred to a centre with an interest in their particular diagnosis. At St George's, avenues like antibiotic and hormone therapies or even vaccines are being explored, increasing the treatment options for some patients. The internet is often a good source of information about what a unit's research interests are and, armed with this information, patients are in a strong position to request a referral from their GP.

Dr Leonard Shapiro

In cardiology, many patients are failing to check that the consultant treating them has sufficient experience, says Dr Leonard Shapiro, Director of Cardiac Services at Papworth Hospital in Cambridge. 'To get the best out of the system you need to be treated by doctors who do a large enough volume of work in this area.'

For consultant cardiologists performing relatively common procedures, such as coronary angiography and coronary angioplasty, there are now clear recommendations as to the level of experience and regular caseload that both the individual operator and the unit should have. And there is a large body of evidence to suggest that patients treated by specialists who meet these recommendations have better outcomes. 'The questions you have to ask your specialist are, "Do you undertake this procedure on a regular basis? How many have you done? Do you specialise solely in this area or is your expertise more general?" For example, in coronary angioplasty, where there are guidelines relating to how many cases should be done by each individual, it would be important to ask, "Do you achieve this number of cases per year?" Evidence suggests that unless you do, you are likely to have less satisfactory outcomes, particularly in the more complex cases.'

The experience of the individual consultant is not the only factor that patients should consider before going forward for procedures like coronary angioplasty. Researchers in the USA have found that the number of operations performed by the unit as a whole also has an impact on outcomes. This may be because in high-volume units, the whole service is more closely tailored to meet the needs of patients with a 'specific problem'. 'If you go to a low-volume operator in a high-volume unit, you are likely to have a satisfactory outcome,' says Shapiro. 'But of course you would be better off with a high-volume operator in the same unit.'

Armed with this evidence, heart services are now being concentrated at fewer, more specialised centres like Papworth Hospital, which treats patients with more complex problems from a wide area. 'We've only got a small number of diseases to deal with,' says Shapiro, 'compared with a district general hospital, where they are also looking after people with strokes, overdoses, broken legs and so on. This enables us to offer patients specialist care from staff who have specific training. That's why we achieved a very favourable CHI [Commission for Health Improvement] report.'

Papworth Hospital is also a research centre, and Shapiro and colleagues are at the forefront of developing techniques for correcting heart disease without the need for open heart surgery. 'I'm an interventional cardiologist, which means I pass fine tubes into the heart to open up valves or arteries, or to repair holes in the heart. I've developed particular expertise in closing holes in the hearts of adults, which prevents them from needing open heart surgery. This technique means that the patient needs only 24 hours in hospital compared to open heart surgery, which requires around seven days' inpatient care.'

Shapiro predicts that as cardiology advances, an increasing proportion of heart operations will be performed by interventional cardiologists, and open heart surgery will become a relatively unusual procedure. This can already be seen in coronary artery disease, where angioplasty is now performed more frequently than bypass surgery.

Another of Shapiro's areas of interest is in the management of athletes with heart disease, and he serves as a medical adviser to the Football Association (FA). Concerns over sudden death from heart disease in athletes have led Shapiro, along with the Football Association and Professional Footballers' Association (PFA), to set up a large-scale screening programme for footballers.

Whether or not you play for Arsenal, however, Shapiro's advice is the same: if you want the best treatment, it is vital to ensure that you are seen at an established centre by a specialist who performs the recommended volume of procedures.

Professor Ken Taylor

The general standard of heart surgery in the UK is very high, and for routine procedures the vast majority of operators do an excellent job, says Professor Ken Taylor, the British Heart Foundation Professor of Cardiac Surgery at Hammersmith Hospital, Imperial College and the University of London. 'I do think that the nature of the UK training programme for cardiothoracic surgeons ensures that when someone finally gets their end-of-training certificate, they are highly experienced in the broad areas of cardiothoracic surgery,' he says.

Taylor concedes that there are some variations, but he thinks that it is really only patients requiring particularly complex or unusual operations who need to concern themselves with their surgeon's special interests. 'There are a number of consultants who have developed, either deliberately or by chance, expertise in specific areas, and that's where patients may seek recommendations for particular individuals.'

One area of a hospital's heart services that is worth considering, however, is how closely integrated the cardiology and cardiac surgery departments are, as Taylor believes that at his own hospital, the Hammersmith, a close working relationship between these specialties has delivered benefits to patients. 'When our workload was expanded several years ago, we deliberately brought the cardiology coronary care unit and the cardiac surgery intensive care unit geographically into the same area of the hospital, where they had common nursing and technical support staff,' he says. 'The closeness of this relationship is very good because it means that a patient coming in with heart disease will not just be going to a cardiologist or a cardiac surgeon, but will be coming to a department where they will be jointly managed.'

This is useful because patients are often transferred between cardiology and cardiac surgery, and in an integrated set-up, the process is easier. 'For many patients, cardiac surgery is not the best initial option,' says Taylor. 'But for those patients who need to be transferred from cardiology investigation or treatment to cardiac surgery, the speed of transfer works very well when you have got an integrated unit, as we have.'

Patients at the Hammersmith also benefit from its academic activities, which in heart surgery have revolved around improving the effectiveness of heart–lung bypass machines. These machines are used in forms of heart surgery where the patient's own heart has to be stopped. Blood is diverted to the machine, which takes over the role of pumping it around the body. The problem has been that the machines are not quite as effective as the natural heart and lungs at supplying oxygen and removing wastes, and they also sometimes cause a harmful inflammatory response. Taylor and his colleagues have been working to minimise these effects through the use of drugs and improvements to the design of the machines themselves, and their progress has translated rapidly into improvements in clinical practice.

'It is why the Hammersmith as an institution was established,' says Taylor, 'to combine the best of clinical research with the best of clinical practice. So that in addition to providing very high quality clinical care, discoveries that were coming out of the research programme could be implemented into the clinical protocol. And I think that formula has worked very well.'

The Hammersmith is also known for its research into heart valves. The UK Heart Valve Registry was established at the hospital in 1986, and has been collecting data on how all of the artificial heart valves that have been implanted since then are performing. The reports the registry publishes help doctors elsewhere to decide which is the best valve to use in a given situation. 'A few months ago, we registered our one hundredth valve prosthesis,' says Taylor. 'It gives us tremendous power in looking for trends, and we are recognised worldwide in terms of the accuracy and completeness of our data.'

Initiatives like the Heart Valve Registry are providing an evidence base to drive improvements in future heart surgery, and Taylor thinks that there will be significant changes in the next few years. In particular, minimally invasive techniques like balloon angioplasty will reduce the need for heart surgery in routine cases of coronary artery disease, and heart surgeons will be freed up to develop surgical options in other conditions, such as heart failure.

Mr Stephen Westaby

Stephen Westaby is the senior adult and paediatric cardiac surgeon at John Radcliffe Hospital in Oxford, with a daily caseload that includes complex heart operations such as repairing damaged heart valves, replacing the diseased aorta and correcting congenital heart defects. He is best known, however, for his pioneering work on mechanical heart pumps, which are almost alone in offering hope to the thousands of people who suffer heart failure in the UK each year.

Westaby became interested in the use of mechanical pumps to treat heart failure during his training in the USA. For people whose heart failure could not be controlled with drugs, the only option was a transplant. But with a chronic shortage of donor hearts and variable outcomes following the operation, their overall outlook was limited. 'I decided that cardiac transplantation simply wasn't going to be the answer, and that we needed new, more realistic, user-friendly devices to solve the heart failure problem,' he says.

Early artificial hearts were large, cumbersome devices that confined the patient to their hospital bed and had to be removed after a limited time. But a major step forward occurred in 1994 when Westaby met US engineer Robert Jarvik and persuaded him to establish a research programme in Oxford to refine a new miniaturised blood pump. After almost ten years of research, this collaboration produced the Jarvik 2000, a device small enough to remain inside the patient indefinitely. 'The research work led to clinical implants, and the Jarvik 2000 is now a very successful device for permanent mechanical circulatory support, and is emerging as an alternative to cardiac transplantation,' Westaby says.

The pump is inserted into the left ventricle, the chamber of the heart that supplies blood to the whole body. It is powered by an external battery pack that plugs in via a socket in the patient's head. This system for power delivery was developed at Oxford, and has significantly reduced the number of infections that patients suffer due to the power cable. Because of funding issues, only a small number of pumps have been implanted in the UK, but the results are promising, and Westaby now hopes to expand their use.

'What we're hoping to do now, having demonstrated on a small number of human implants that the device is safe and very effective, is a prospective randomised trial of the Jarvik 2000 versus continued conventional medical treatment,' he says. For this, Westaby is in the process of applying to the Department of Health for funding. Until now, all of the work done on the device has been funded by a research grant and money from charities.

One of the most encouraging things to emerge from the work done so far on artificial heart pumps has been the discovery that a failing heart can recover if it is supported by a pump and allowed to rest. Westaby is now exploring the cellular and molecular mechanisms for this recovery, which he hopes may lead to the discovery of new and more effective drugs for treating heart failure.

'The most exciting phenomenon in this programme is where we have rested end-stage failing hearts with a blood pump and they have got a lot better,' he says. 'What we and others have found is that when hearts go into failure, their genes go back into the same configuration as in the foetus. Resting the heart brings back the normal configuration. I am now working on elucidating the molecular mechanism of how the heart muscle recovers when it is rested. Using these pathways, we may be able to trick the heart into thinking it has a pump when it hasn't. That way we'll be able to treat the patients a lot earlier and hopefully prevent the heart failure progressing before the stage where they need either a transplant or a pump.'

While artificial heart pumps are an exciting area of research, the bulk of Westaby's surgical work is more conventional heart surgery. He performs several hundred difficult heart operations a year, often on high-risk patients referred to him from other parts of the UK and overseas. 'I actually operate on a full spectrum of patients, from premature infants all the way through to people in their nineties,' he says.

He strongly believes that patients who are in need of a complex operation should check their surgeon's record in the area, as different individuals' outcomes for the same procedure can vary dramatically, even within the same hospital. 'All cardiac surgeons have certain weaknesses, and one of those weaknesses is often overestimating the scope of their capabilities,' he says. 'A surgeon will always tell you he's got great experience, but at the end of the day, you find out what people are really interested in by looking them up on the internet.'

The internet can contain a lot of extraneous information, so it is important to know what you are looking for. For surgeons, the best indicator of surgical skill is that they have published their results for a particular operation in a respected medical journal. Westaby believes this sort of information is a better indicator than more general mortality figures, which do not always account for the complexity of the surgery performed or the sickness of the patient. 'League tables relate only to coronary bypass. This is operating on the surface of the heart, and from my perspective it is not an index of how good a cardiac surgeon you are. Surgeons can choose their patients sufficiently well to achieve a 100 per cent survival rate. The coronary artery results might be good, but their abilities to operate within the heart may be limited,' he says.

Similarly, cardiologists are not necessarily the best source of information about who is a good cardiac surgeon because they often have close links with individual surgeons through private practice. Despite these difficulties, Westaby thinks that patients should make an effort to find out about their surgeon before the consultation. 'A lot of patients come and have no real concept of what to ask. They haven't checked out the expertise of the surgeon, and you start off on the wrong foot if you launch in with, "Well how many of these have you done before?"' he says. 'I think the best time to check your surgeon's credentials is before you ever get near him.'

Parkinson's disease

What is the specialty?

Neurology and medicine for the elderly.

What is Parkinson's disease?

Parkinson's disease is a progressive neurological disorder that affects movement, muscle control and balance. It is named after Dr James Parkinson (1755–1824), the London doctor who first identified Parkinson's as a specific condition. There is no cure, but drugs can be effective in relieving symptoms. There are three main symptoms of the disease.

- Akinesia describes the difficulty people with Parkinson's often find in initiating, performing and sustaining coordinated movements and accounts for their lack of facial expression, small, cramped writing and low-volume monotonous speech. Bradykinesia means slowness of movement.
- Rigidity and stiffness of the limbs, trunk and neck.
- Tremor or shaking of the limbs, tongue or jaw. In the hand, tremors are more pronounced when at rest or when the patient is under stress. About 70 per cent of patients have a tremor.

Other symptoms of the disease can include unsteadiness, difficulty in walking, tiredness, depression, problems with sexual and bladder function, constipation and, in a minority, dementia. Dementia develops in 30 per cent of older patients and resembles Alzheimer's disease. Symptoms usually begin slowly and on one side, and develop gradually, in no particular order. The rate of development and severity of the symptoms are very individual and vary from patient to patient. They become more pronounced as the disease progresses, and patients ultimately experience difficulty with simple tasks such as walking and speaking. However, it can take years before symptoms develop to a point where they cause major problems. Other conditions can mimic the symptoms of Parkinson's, and it can be a side-effect of some drugs. As there are no accurate blood tests available that can confirm the presence of the disease, misdiagnosis is common (see Brooks, p.166; Clarke, p.171; Lees and Quinn, p.175).

The exact cause of Parkinson's is unknown, although a few genes that cause it are now identified. The disease comes about when over half of the dopamine cells in the brain are destroyed. Dopamine works in balance with another chemical called acetylcholine to transmit messages between nerve cells and muscles, and these messages enable us to perform a range of movements. In people with Parkinson's, this balance is upset by the loss of dopamine cells.

What are the statistics?
Around 100,000 people in the UK – one in 600 – have Parkinson's disease. Symptoms usually appear after the age of 50, and the risk of getting the disease increases with age. Most sufferers of Parkinson's are over the age of 70, and men are affected slightly more often than women. About 10,000 people in the UK are diagnosed each year, and in one in twenty of these, symptoms will have started before the age of 40, when it is known as young-onset Parkinson's disease. It is estimated that four million people worldwide have Parkinson's.

How is it currently treated?
There is no cure for Parkinson's disease. However, there are a number of effective treatments that can minimise the symptoms of the disease and maximise quality of life. The most common treatment is either Sinemet, which is a combination of the drugs levodopa and carbidopa, or Madopar, which is a combination of the drugs levodopa and benserazide.

Levodopa is a dopamine precursor, a substance that is transformed into dopamine by the brain. The introduction of levodopa in the 1970s revolutionised treatment for Parkinson's. Before it came on the market there was no effective treatment for patients with the disease, and it has remained the most successful drug available today. Levodopa is always prescribed in combination with either carbidopa or benserazide, as these drugs stop levodopa from being metabolised by the body and allow more of it to get to the brain. The advantage too is that a smaller dose of levodopa is needed to treat symptoms, and certain unpleasant side-effects, which include nausea and vomiting, are greatly reduced. There is very little difference between carbidopa and benserazide, and their use varies from country to country. Both combinations of these drugs are available and widely prescribed in the UK, while the USA only has Sinemet and eastern Europe, Madopar.

One of the drawbacks of levodopa as a treatment is that over time patients can develop fluctuations in motor response to the drug and abnormal involuntary movements called dyskinesias. After one year's treatment, 10 per cent of patients will develop dyskinesias and after five years 50 per cent of patients will have developed them. Younger patients are more prone to these complications – after five years on levodopa-based drugs over 80 per cent will have developed them. There is also a form of the disease prevalent among some ethnic minority groups that is resistant to levodopa therapy (see Chaudhuri, p.170).

The most effective alternative treatment to levodopa is dopamine agonists. These are a class of drugs that activate the dopamine receptors directly. They can be taken alone or in combination with levodopa-based drugs. On their own, dopamine agonists can delay the onset of motor complications, but these drugs are not as effective as levodopa. Dopamine agonists have a greater tendency than levodopa to cause nausea, vomiting and hallucinations. Side-effects are more pronounced in older patients.

Because of the problems associated with levodopa, younger people with Parkinson's now often start with dopamine agonists, reserving levodopa for a later stage of the disease. Older patients are generally started with levodopa. However, there is currently much debate over which type of drug should be used as a first treatment for Parkinson's in older patients, and trials are currently taking place in the UK to examine this issue.

Other treatment options are enzyme inhibitors. The COMT inhibitor entacapone, taken in conjunction with levodopa, prolongs its effects by blocking the action of an enzyme which breaks down levodopa before it reaches the brain. Selegiline, a MAOB inhibitor, blocks an enzyme which breaks down dopamine. Amantadine is a drug which has mild anti-parkinsonian effects in early Parkinson's disease, but can reduce levodopa-induced involuntary movements later in the disease. Anticholinergic drugs, such as benzhexol, can have useful anti-tremor effect in young patients with early disease, but can cause confusion in older patients, in whom they are usually avoided.

Surgery is another important treatment in late-stage patients. Prior to the discovery of levodopa, surgery was the only treatment option for some people with Parkinson's disease. In the last few decades, surgery has gained new popularity. Thalamic surgery only helps tremor and rigidity, not akinesia or dyskinesias. Pallidal surgery mainly helps dyskinesias.

The main form of surgery that is now used for patients with Parkinson's disease is deep brain stimulation (DBS) of the subthalamic nuclei, which improves most features of Parkinson's disease and also enables drug dosages to be decreased, with a consequent reduction in drug-induced involuntary movements.

How does that measure up to treatment in the rest of Europe and the USA?

Parkinson's patients in the UK have access to all available drugs on the market. So long as diagnosis and prescribing are overseen by a neurologist or geriatrician with a particular interest in Parkinson's disease, then patient care is as good as anywhere in the world. Access to surgery remains limited, however. Deep brain stimulation technology is expensive: its cost-effectiveness is currently being assessed in a national trial randomising patients to surgery (usually implantation of DBS) or best medical treatment before the NHS is prepared to fund it routinely as an approved treatment for selected cases. In many European countries and the USA, patients have access to only one levodopa combination drug (Sinemet or Madopar), whereas the UK has both available.

An issue for patients in the UK is in the delay in getting to see a consultant. The UK has the lowest number of neurologists per head of population in the developed world. There are only around 200 consultant neurologists in the UK, whereas most European countries have five times the UK propotion and the USA ten times that propotion (see Chaudhuri, p.169).

The low consultant–patient ratio is reflected in how long Parkinson's patients in the UK can spend with their consultants. Outpatient appointments for new patients may only be 20 to 30 minutes long, while follow-up appointments are often no longer than ten minutes. The Association of British Neurologists has suggested that 40 minutes should be allocated to new patients and

20 minutes for follow-up appointments (see Chaudhuri, p.169; Lees and Quinn, p.176).

However, the low number of consultant neurologists is offset by the use of Parkinson's disease nurse specialists in many clinics around the country. These nurses are promoted by the Parkinson's Disease Society (PDS) and work alongside consultants in their clinics. They see patients after their appointment with the consultant, giving them time to ask additional questions and making sure that they understand the issues. They sometimes conduct their own clinic lists alongside consultants. They are essential for the initiation of treatment with subcutaneous apomorphine injections or infusion. Nurses also provide follow-up care in the community. There are currently around 100 Parkinson's disease nurses in the UK. The PDS aims to increase this number to 240, so that there is one nurse per health region, giving reasonable coverage across the country (see Findley, p.174).

What new treatments are available?

There are no new classes of drugs for Parkinson's disease that have recently come on to the market, but there are a number of drugs in the early stages of development.

Can I get these on the NHS?

All drugs that are on the market for Parkinson's disease are available on the NHS. It is likely that as new drugs come on the market, these also will be available on the NHS so long as they are found by the National Institute for Clinical Excellence (NICE) to be clinically and cost effective, and safe.

What treatments are in the pipeline?

A number of promising new drugs are being evaluated for Parkinson's disease, but all are in very early stages of development and are unlikely to be licensed for at least five years. The closest to the market are dopamine agonists that are administered in the form of a patch rather than a pill, for continuous stimulation.

Other experimental treatments are a long way off being available to patients, and much more research is needed. Some research into Parkinson's disease involves implanting cells or infusing growth factors into the brain. One pilot study that shows promise involves infusing glial derived neurotrophic factor (GDNF) into a specific part of the brain. A few patients so far studied in a British trial, led by Stephen Gill, a neurosurgeon at Frenchay Hospital in Bristol, have experienced improvements in their symptoms, but further controlled studies are needed (see Brooks, p.167).

Another important study involved injecting retinal cells into the brain. These cells, normally found at the back of the eye, produce dopamine. Researchers at Emory University, Atlanta, discovered that, after a year, the coordination and motor control of Parkinson's disease patients had improved. However, the results of these two trials are preliminary, and it is too soon to say how long the benefits may last or whether the treatments could be used on other patients.

Transplants of human and porcine foetal brain tissue are also being researched, but there are obvious ethical problems (see Brooks, p.168). These may be overcome by using stem cells produced by cloning techniques. Stem cells are embryonic cells or adult cells that have the potential to develop into some of the cell types found in the body. Researchers have taken advanced stem cells from rats and made them develop into dopamine-producing brain cells, which survived for two weeks in mouse brains. However, human trials of stem cell grafting are still two to five years away. There are potential dangers with cell implantation into the brain. At least two patients have died from overgrowth producing a cyst or a tumour. Also, some patients who have received foetal cell grafts have subsequently developed troublesome dyskinesias.

Another large trial (PD SURG) will look at the effectiveness and cost of several new surgical treatments for Parkinson's. The main technique under scrutiny is deep brain stimulation, and the trial will compare outcomes for patients who have surgery at a much earlier stage to outcomes for those who wait for the normal length of time (see Clarke, p.172).

Who treats it?

If your GP suspects you may have Parkinson's disease, you should be referred to a neurologist or a geriatrician, preferably with a particular interest in Parkinson's disease, to confirm the diagnosis and formulate a treatment plan. Your specialist will send details of any treatment you need to your GP, who will coordinate your care, give you advice and information, organise any occupational therapy and prescribe your medication. However, your consultant will continuously assess the progression of the disease and your response to the treatment plan, which may change accordingly.

There are no laboratory tests that can be used accurately to diagnose Parkinson's disease (but see Brooks, p.166; Lees and Quinn, p.175). Diagnosis relies on clinical experience and, as the symptoms mimic other conditions, it is very important that you be referred to a specialist Parkinson's neurologist or geriatrician for diagnosis (see Brooks, p.167; Clarke, p.171).

What training will the specialist have?

Before becoming a consultant, your doctor will have had a general medical training, which includes five years at university followed by one year as a House Officer, before gaining registration with the General Medical Council. They will then have spent two to three years as a Senior House Officer in various medical disciplines. This is followed by a five- or six-year period of specialist registrar training in neurology, working in different hospitals, leading to a Certificate of Completion of Specialist Training that is recognised throughout Europe. In the fifth year and post-certification, doctors are encouraged to train to become sub-specialists. It is preferable for Parkinson's disease patients to see a consultant neurologist or geriatrician with a special interest in Parkinson's disease, as they will be an expert in this area.

Where will I receive care?

You will first see your neurologist or geriatrician as an outpatient at the hospital or clinic from which they work. Outpatient departments are non-ward areas, and you will see your consultant in a private room.

What questions should I ask about my treatment?

Write down a list of questions to ask your consultant about your treatment and take them with you to your first outpatient's appointment. Take a family member with you and ask them to write down consultant responses. Questions might include:

- What treatments are available?
- Which is the best treatment for me?
- What can I expect to get from the treatment?
- When is it going to work?
- How long am I going to be on it?
- Are there any side-effects?
- What is the short-term prognosis?
- What is the long-term prognosis?
- Are there any new trials that I can be involved in?
- If so, what are the risks?

What will my treatment involve?

Your first appointment will last for between 15 and 30 minutes, and during this time your consultant will confirm your diagnosis, assess the degree of disability, set a treatment plan in place and answer any questions you have. If your consultant has a Parkinson's disease specialist nurse assisting at their clinic, you may then be seen by them. Your nurse will provide support, counselling and follow-up care, alongside your GP.

Most of your care will be carried out in the community under the direction of your GP. Your consultant will usually write to your GP and give detailed advice on what drugs to prescribe. If you respond well to the treatment, you will see your consultant again within three months. If not, you will see your consultant sooner, and they will adjust your dose accordingly. Whenever you need a new drug treatment plan your GP will refer you back to your consultant.

What makes a REAL difference to getting better?

As there is no cure for Parkinson's disease, treatment focuses on reducing the symptoms of the disease and increasing quality of life. The best quality of care for Parkinson's disease comes not just from the best use of drugs but from getting the diagnosis right in the first place. Studies have shown that the error rate for diagnosis from GPs is 51 per cent, compared with just 10 per cent for Parkinson's specialists. Once the diagnosis is correct, then drug treatment becomes critical and changes according to the progression of the disease and the response to the treatment plan. Therefore, from a diagnostic point of view and a treatment point of view, the most critical treatment factor for people with Parkinson's disease is that they see an expert in the condition. It is also beneficial to patients to be seen by a consultant who works alongside a specialist Parkinson's nurse, as you will receive more follow-up care. To ensure you receive the best possible care you should receive:

- diagnosis from an expert
- a treatment plan from an expert
- care from a consultant who has a Parkinson's specialist nurse.

What is the difference between a well-run and a badly run clinic?

A good Parkinson's clinic will be run by a consultant who is a specialist in Parkinson's disease, rather than just a general neurologist or geriatrician. At a good clinic, consultants will be supported by specialist Parkinson's disease nurses, who follow up patients both at the surgery and once they have returned home. A lack of facilities for occupational therapy is not necessarily the mark of a badly run clinic, as these can be accessed in the community under the care of your GP.

Will I get better treatment if I go privately?

The most important aspect of your treatment is that it is overseen by a specialist who has a particular interest in Parkinson's disease. Many consultants work in the private sector as well as the NHS, so it is possible to see a specialist neurologist both publicly and privately. The main benefit to seeking private care is that you bypass waiting lists and will have more time with a specialist during your consultations. In the private sector some neurologists divide their initial consultations into two separate sittings, so that the patient has time to digest the information and ask about issues that have cropped up since the first discussion. Consultants rarely have time to do this in the NHS. Another benefit of private care is that you are likely to receive more physiotherapy, which is an important part of the treatment plan for Parkinson's.

Will I get better treatment if I go abroad?

Parkinson's patients in the UK have access to all available drugs on the market and all surgical techniques. So long as diagnosis and prescribing is overseen by a neurologist or geriatrician with a particular interest in Parkinson's disease, then patient care in the UK is just as good as anywhere in the world.

What support will I be offered by the clinic and are there any independent support groups I can join?

The level of support you will be offered depends on the facilities of the unit or hospital, but most additional support, such as occupational therapy, is carried out in the community under the direction of your GP. Some clinics have specialist Parkinson's nurses who will provide additional support and counselling. Ask your GP what facilities the unit has when he or she refers you to a consultant.

The Parkinson's Disease Society (PDS) is a good independent source of help and advice. They organise support groups around the country and can put you in touch with a group in your area.

Useful addresses

The European Parkinson's Disease Association
EPDA Liaison/Project Manager
4 Golding Road
Sevenoaks
Kent TN13 3NJ
Tel 01732 457683
Email: admin@epda.eu.com
www.shef.ac.uk/~nr1pp/test/

Parkinson's Disease Society
215 Vauxhall Bridge Road
London SW1V 1EJ
Tel 020 7931 8080
Helpline 0808 800 0303 (9.30 am to 5.30 pm Monday to Friday)
www.parkinsons.org.uk.

Expert opinions

Professor David Brooks

The first problem in the treatment of Parkinson's disease is working out which patients actually have the illness, as it is easily confused with a number of other conditions. Getting this right can be crucial in identifying the right treatment.

Professor David Brooks is one of the UK's leading experts in movement disorders such as Parkinson's disease, tremors and dystonia. He works at the Medical Research Council's Clinical Science Centre at Hammersmith Hospital in London, where the focus of research is on using new techniques to better diagnose and understand Parkinson's.

By using a sophisticated system of scanning the brain, he has found that as many as 10 per cent of new Parkinson's patients have been misdiagnosed. The technique he uses is called positron emission tomography (PET) scanning. In contrast to other imaging techniques, such as magnetic resonance imaging (MRI) and computerised tomography (CT), which can reveal the structure of the brain, PET scanning provides information on how the brain is working. The technique relies on taking a natural substance, such as glucose, making it mildly radioactive for an hour or two, and injecting it into the patient. Using a scanner, doctors can then map out where the substance ends up in the body.

In Parkinson's disease, damage typically occurs to a system of nerves called dopamine nerves in the brain. These take in a simple substance called dopa and convert it into dopamine, a process that can be monitored using radioactive dopa and PET. 'You can see the dopa being taken up and changed into dopamine by the dopamine nerves,' says Brooks, 'So it's a way of looking at how the nerves function.'

'If people come to us with a diagnosis of Parkinson's, in many cases it will be fairly clear-cut clinically. But there are a group of patients where you're not really sure. In those situations, it can be very useful to do a scan to determine whether their dopamine nerves are working properly.'

'We've now done two large trials where people sent us newly diagnosed, untreated cases,' he says. 'What has emerged is about a 10 per cent discordance. Ten per cent of the people sent to us didn't have Parkinson's disease on their scans, even though they had been labelled as such.' This 10 per cent discordance was for patients referred by specialists, and it is possible that the discordance for people diagnosed by GPs is even greater.

For people showing early signs of Parkinson's disease, the priority must be for them to see a specialist as early as possible. 'The first thing the patient needs is to get to a clinician who understands their condition. A lot of patients are still managed by their GPs alone. Probably only half of elderly patients with Parkinson's disease get to see a specialist right at the beginning,' he says.

If they don't see a specialist, Parkinson's patients are usually prescribed an L-dopa preparation for the condition. But this can lead to difficulties in the long term. 'One of the problems with the standard treatment of Parkinson's is that three or four years down the line you start to get into complications from the drugs,' says Brooks. 'Most of us are now trying to use different ways of treating the disease initially to avoid these complications.'

Even patients who do see a neurologist have no guarantee that they are seeing a specialist with a particular interest in their condition. 'Many neurologists like to see a bit of everything to get variety, and are rather reluctant to send patients to specialist clinics,' says Brooks. 'The first thing the patient should really ask is, "Do you have a particular interest in this condition?" and if not, "Is there someone among your group of neurologists who does?" Most big neuroscience centres will now tell you what their various neurologists are particularly interested in, and you should, without offending anybody, be able to be sent to the relevant clinic.'

In addition to holding general neurology clinics and specialist clinics in movement disorders, Brooks is involved in frontline neurological research. 'One of the things I'm particularly interested in is trying to work out whether transplants or transfusing nerve growth factors directly into the brain can reverse degenerative diseases and restore brain function again,' he says.

In one trial at Frenchay Hospital in Bristol, a nerve growth factor called glial derived neurotrophic factor (GDNF) has been transfused directly into the brains of Parkinson's patients. 'The results have been quite striking,' says Brooks. 'Within a few weeks patients are extremely improved, and PET scans have shown an increase in their dopamine function. It looks as if this growth factor is probably having a wide range of actions, not just on the dopamine nerves but on other brain nerves as well. It's looking a very interesting and promising approach.'

Transplants could also offer significant benefits to Parkinson's sufferers. 'If you put cells from a human foetus, which come from the part of the brain called the mid-brain, into a Parkinson's patient, they get dramatically better,' he says. 'The big problem is how you make this a practical reality for the general patient. What we have to do now is produce a large cell culture, rather like a pot of yoghurt, where you can just produce these cells to order without the need for foetuses, which has emotional and ethical problems.'

While these advances are a source of hope for Parkinson's sufferers, they are still some way from reaching the frontline of treatment. The current priority for patients is to get the right diagnosis and drug regimen, and the best way to do this is to see a specialist in movement disorders as early as possible.

Dr K Ray Chaudhuri

In some parts of the country patients with Parkinson's disease are not receiving the full range of treatment options available because of a shortage of specialists and the high cost of the drugs involved, says Dr K. Ray Chaudhuri, a consultant neurologist at both King's College Hospital and Lewisham Hospital in London. At the heart of the problem is a national shortage of neurologists. At the moment, the UK has one neurologist per 177,000 people, which is significantly fewer than many European countries. In comparison France, for example, has one neurologist per 38,500 people, a considerable diference.

With overcrowded clinics and an increasing number of drugs available to treat conditions like Parkinson's, it is inevitable that patients are not discussing the full range of options. 'If you are really stretched and you have got lots of patients waiting, each patient is only going to get 10 or 15 minutes in your clinic,' says Chaudhuri. 'That is hardly any time, and people then get put on the easiest option, which is levodopa. Very often I am seeing people who have just been told they have got Parkinson's disease and that they should start the standard levodopa treatment. If I was a patient, I would want to know what the latest developments are and then make an informed choice myself.'

Levodopa has been the standard treatment for Parkinson's for many years, and is a cheap and effective drug in many cases. Unfortunately, its usefulness in controlling the disease declines over time, and some patients start to develop movement problems from the drug itself after prolonged use. For these reasons, many experts are now using newer drugs, such as dopamine agonists, to control the disease in its early stages. 'One has to remember that about 40 or 50 per cent of people starting on levodopa will develop abnormal movement in four or five years' time,' says Chaudhuri. 'If the patient says, "Look, I want a quick effect and I don't care about what happens in four or five years' time," then sure, they can go on levodopa. But at least they should be give the choice. In my hands, certainly, all the younger ones first go on an agonist treatment, and most of them have done very well.'

More studies are needed before doctors will be able to say definitively what is the best way to treat Parkinson's in its early stages. However, for NHS patients the debate is often coloured by issues of cost, as the newer drugs can be very expensive. 'There is an increasing conflict with our hospital managers, because as the condition becomes more recognised and treatable, the cost of treatment is rising, and so cost-effectiveness issues are becoming increasingly important.'

Standard drug therapy can be particularly inappropriate for Parkinson's patients from some ethnic minority groups, where a form of the disease that is resistant to levodopa therapy is particularly prevalent. This is one of Chaudhuri's main areas of interest. 'What we have found is that there is a certain subset of first-generation African-Caribbean immigrants who have a form of Parkinson's that is relatively resistant to levodopa treatment. The proportion of these resistant people is three times higher than for white Caucasians. The problem is if the doctor is not aware of this, people can often just be told that they may not have Parkinson's disease, or that they are resistant to the drugs and nothing is going to work. In fact, they might just need an increased dosage of the same drug.'

In the future, Chaudhuri hopes to develop an 'ethnicity package' for Parkinson's that will offer guidance to doctors treating patients from the target groups. Similar initiatives already exist in other areas, such as diabetes and high blood pressure.

At present, the best way around these problems is to get to a Parkinson's specialist at a dedicated clinic, but this can be very difficult in some parts of the UK. 'What's happening is a lot of postcode prescribing,' he says. 'If you're in some areas of the UK, you are unlikely to see a Parkinson's specialist or a specialist nurse, whereas in most parts of London you will get that.'

With clinics sparsely distributed and oversubscribed, some Parkinson's patients face an uphill struggle to get to see a specialist. This, together with pressure to reduce costs, means that at present, patients must be wary of starting the standard levodopa therapy without sufficient discussion of the alternatives.

Dr Carl Clarke

Dr Carl Clarke, a clinical neurology specialist at Birmingham's City Hospital, recently saw a patient who had been living with a diagnosis of Parkinson's disease for the last 17 years, and told him that he had never had the condition. This highlights a serious problem for Parkinson's patients nationwide. Too often the condition is being misdiagnosed by doctors without sufficient expertise. 'There was a study done a couple of years ago in Wales showing that the error rate in general practice is about 50 per cent,' he says.

The problem is not limited to GPs. Studies carried out retrospectively on the brains of Parkinson's sufferers after they have died reveal that general neurologists and general geriatricians have an error rate of around 25 per cent – one quarter of the patients they diagnose with Parkinson's turn out not to have the condition. Clarke's own patient had been to see two hospital specialists during the time he was misdiagnosed as a Parkinson's sufferer, and neither spotted the problem. Clarke is quick to point out that this does not reflect on their ability; it is just that their interests lay elsewhere.

'Take those two doctors who saw the patient,' he says. 'If I had a different condition called neuropathy, I would unequivocally go to one of them, who is quite an authority – certainly the best in the area. And if I had a serious head injury or a member of my family was comatose, I would go to the other guy. I wouldn't come to me instead. It is all to do with sub-specialisation within neurology.'

The problem centres on the fact that there are no truly diagnostic tests for Parkinson's disease, and it can closely resemble other more common conditions such as essential tremor, which is what Clarke's patient turned out to have. Making the correct diagnosis, then, depends heavily on the experience of the individual specialist.

Clarke thinks that the best way to ensure that the specialist you are seeing is an expert is to check that they are running a specialist movement disorders clinic and that they have done a research degree, and MD or PhD, in the area. Patients are best not diagnosed by GPs or general neurologists, and certainly treatment should not be started until a specialist has been consulted, as the standard drugs for Parkinson's, such as levodopa, can cause irreversible problems in people who take them over a long period of time – whether they actually have Parkinson's or not.

It is important for patients to check their consultant's interests themselves, as GPs do not always know where the specialist clinics are held. 'I've advertised the service myself,' says Clarke, 'but GPs get so much junk mail, and neurology is not quite top of their – or the Government's – agenda, so it doesn't always register.'

Clarke's research interests centre on setting up large-scale trials to evaluate new techniques for treating Parkinson's. In one of these, the PD MED trial, they hope to recruit thousands of Parkinson's patients, with both early- and late-stage disease, and put them on either levodopa or one of the newer drugs. The patients will then be followed up for five to ten years, and researchers will compare the outcomes, quality of life and economics of the treatments in the hope of producing a set of guidelines governing their use.

Another large trial, the PD SURG trial, will look at the effectiveness and cost of several new surgical treatments for Parkinson's. The main technique under scrutiny is deep brain stimulation, in which a pacemaker system is implanted into a small area deep within the brain. When the electrical current is switched on, the area of the brain around the implant is effectively over-stimulated and switched off, which can produce dramatic improvements in the condition of the patient.

Surgical interventions like deep brain stimulation are currently only used in patients who can no longer be treated effectively with drugs, and the waiting time at most centres is 12 to 18 months. The PD SURG trial will compare outcomes for patients who have surgery at a much earlier stage to outcomes for those who wait for the normal length of time. 'There are a huge number of unanswered questions here which we need answered before the Government starts investing millions of pounds on this treatment,' says Clarke.

These two large trials are likely to provide neurologists with a better idea of how to treat Parkinson's in the next few years. However, the major problem facing patients today is establishing whether they suffer from the disease at all. And with error rates for diagnosis as high as 50 per cent in general practice, it is essential that they seek a specialist's opinion before commencing treatment.

Professor Leslie Findley

The aspects of Parkinson's disease that most affect sufferers' quality of life are being overlooked by many specialists in the condition, says Professor Leslie Findley, an eminent neurologist based at the Essex Neuroscience Unit at Oldchurch Hospital.

Findley recently coordinated a landmark global survey into Parkinson's disease, asking suffers for their views on the condition and its treatment. The results showed that depression was the single most important influence on quality of life, more significant than disease severity or medication. 'Emotional and psychological factors are, to me, responsible for the majority of quality of life, even in the severely affected, and these are often missed,' says Findley. 'Patients will get treated, and their tremors will be reduced or their stiffness removed, but they are still incapacitated in their ability to enjoy and participate in the real world.'

In Findley's view, a good Parkinson's specialist must be someone who is prepared to tackle all aspects of the disease. 'You've really got to go to a doctor who is taking a holistic view on the subject, rather than someone who technically knows all about the latest dopa agonists,' he says.

This is not to underestimate the importance of a high level of sub-specialisation and expertise in the condition, as Parkinson's and similar conditions like essential tremor can be tricky to diagnose. 'In essence, movement disorders are a clinician's joy, because they still rely predominantly on clinical assessment and evaluation. The cardinal sin is to diagnose something that is essential tremor as Parkinson's and then start the patient on medications which have quite potent side-effects, because once the diagnosis has been made, minds tend to close and the patient ends up in the system of repeat prescriptions.'

But as well as expertise, the doctor's manner in dealing with patients is a factor worth considering because, especially around the time of diagnosis, it can have a lasting effect on their attitude to the disease. 'A badly managed diagnostic experience impacts on that patient forever,' says Findley. 'Whatever else happens to them, if they feel they weren't given enough time or information at the point of diagnosis and in the weeks that followed, it influences that patient's quality of life forever. Basically, quality of life derives from coming to terms with the condition and moving on, and if they don't feel they've had a fair crack of the whip at the beginning, then they never really adjust to it.'

There is only a limited amount a consultant can do to help patients come to terms with their diagnosis at the consultation, so this is an area where other specialists, particularly nurses, come into play. In Findley's view, the importance of these expert staff cannot be overstated, and patients should be wary of a Parkinson's service that does not include them. 'These days, a unit without specialist nurse input is going to be a poor unit,' he says. 'As a patient, I would want to know that there was support from a specialist nurse and access to a multi-disciplinary team.'

Findley's unit runs a training programme for specialist Parkinson's nurses, who then go on to operate away from the hospital in the community. This day-to-day involvement with patients provides them with a much better insight into individual problems than the hospital specialist has. 'Once he's made the diagnosis and started treatment, is the consultant going to see the patient for six months? No. Does he know anything about that person's position in the community, their family structure, their relationship with the GP? No. All the other problems, like constipation, sexual problems, pain, all the issues you can think of, which are tedious to doctors, are picked up by the specialist nurse. These nurses are incredibly well trained. They are even taught how to manage doctors, because they are going to have more specific knowledge of the condition than the GP. But they are not there to antagonise the GP, rather to bolster the system and make everyone feel sure.'

Unfortunately, there are still not enough of these specialist nurses – around another 100 are needed nationally to achieve comprehensive coverage. Findley feels that addressing this issue should be a priority in Parkinson's care, as only a partnership between these professionals and specialist doctors can deliver the best possible quality of life to patients.

Professor Andrew Lees
and Professor Niall Quinn

Andrew Lees and Niall Quinn are Professors of Neurology at the National Hospital for Neurology and Neurosurgery at Queen Square in London. The National is one of the world's leading centres for the research and treatment of neurological disorders such as Parkinson's disease, and receives complex referrals from across the country. 'We are the backstop of the service,' says Quinn. 'Where other neurologists get difficult diagnostic cases that they can't make up their mind about, or cases that are proving difficult to treat, they ask us if we can help.'

As well as Parkinson's disease, the centre researches into and treats a range of neurological disorders such as progressive supranuclear palsy (PSP) and multiple system atrophy (MSA), which are often initially misdiagnosed as Parkinson's. They also specialise in other movement disorders such as chorea, tics, myoclonus, tremor and dystonia.

To deal with these conditions, the National brings together a wider range of specialists than a typical neurology service. This is particularly important in treating MSA, which in addition to affecting the motor part of the nervous system also affects the autonomic (or unconscious) nervous system that controls blood pressure and bladder function. 'We are particularly well-placed in relation to MSA because we have a professor of neurovascular medicine, Chris Mathias, whose interest is autonomic failure,' says Quinn. 'We also have the country's only professor of uroneurology, Clare Fowler, who is the expert on the nervous control of the bladder, particularly the Parkinson's bladder. They can help in both diagnosis and management of these atypical patients.' Lees and Quinn are assisted by postgraduate research fellows specialising in movement disorders, and specialist nurses. They also work closely with movement disorder specialists Dr Kailash Bhatia and Dr Patricia Limousin – Dr Limousin assessing patients for possible brain surgery if medications are not controlling their symptoms adequately.

The centre is also equipped with a battery of high-tech equipment for testing and diagnosis. For example, there is a single-photon emission computed tomography (SPECT) scanner, which enables doctors to look directly at how the brain is functioning. Lees points out, however, that in this area no test is a substitute for clinical skill in making a diagnosis. 'The bottom line is that it is the skill of the physician that is needed to dissect out these different conditions, one from the other. The tests are all marginally helpful, but none is so definitive that it will give us a clear answer,' he says.

Patients visiting a tertiary referral centre like the National can be sure that they will be seeing or will be referred on to a leading expert in their condition. What can be more variable in many settings is the amount of time they have with their consultant, and the consultant's ability to communicate with them. 'Good bedside manner is the most important thing,' says Lees. 'Some of the smartest people in medicine have useless bedside skills, and professors generally have a rather bad reputation for that. You need somebody who knows what they are up to but who also sees a lot of patients.'

This is particularly true for Parkinson's, as patients often find it difficult to communicate effectively within the short space of time they have at a consultation. 'The trouble with Parkinson's is that you often need to go into considerable detail to make the correct diagnosis and know how best to modify the patient's treatment,' says Quinn. 'If you have a clinic where the doctor can only spend five or ten minutes with a patient, it is often impossible to make a thorough assessment in such a short space of time.'

Tertiary centres like the National offer a range of specialists and facilities that is suited to the more difficult patients they treat. However, the same basic principles of patient care apply here as much as in any other setting, and Lees and Quinn both stress how important it is that other priorities, such as research and management, do not interfere with this.

Stroke

What is the specialty?

General medicine, medicine for the elderly, stroke medicine or neurology, depending on where you live (see Warlow, p.201).

What is a stroke?

A stroke happens when there is an interruption of blood flow to part of the brain, causing brain cells to die through lack of oxygen. This can lead to paralysis, loss of speech, memory and vision, diminished reasoning, depression or even death. Symptoms depend on which part of the brain has been deprived of blood. There are two main types:

ISCHAEMIC STROKE

This happens when a blood vessel becomes blocked. This most commonly arises from atherosclerosis (furring of the arteries), embolism (circulating blood clots from the heart or large blood vessels) or disease of the small blood vessels in the brain.

HAEMORRHAGIC STROKE

This happens when a weakened blood vessel bursts and blood leaks into the brain causing damage. This type causes more deaths than ischaemic stroke but those who survive it recover more fully.

What are the statistics?

Each year around 120,000 people in England and Wales have a stroke. For around 100,000 this will be a first stroke and for 20,000 it will be a second or subsequent stroke. The vast majority (around 90 per cent) are aged over 55. However, each year around 10,000 people aged under 55 and 1,000 people under 30 have a stroke. Men are more at risk, but because women live longer than men and strokes are more common with increasing age, the total number of strokes is in a ratio of about 60 to 40 women to men. People of African-Caribbean and South Asian origin are more at risk. Stroke is one of the UK's biggest killers, accounting for 12 per cent of deaths or, to put it another way, some 70,000 people each year. Stroke is also the single most common cause of severe disability. Currently, some 300,000 people are living with disabilities caused by a stroke. Once you have had a stroke you are at a high risk of having another one. About one in six people who have had a stroke will go on to have another one within two years. In the UK, stroke is the single most expensive condition to treat.

How is it currently treated?

Before the establishment of the NHS in 1948 there was no specific treatment for stroke. Patients used to be sent to municipal hospitals, where they often languished and died. A big change in attitude came in the 1950s with the introduction of anticoagulants (clot-thinning drugs), a spin-off from research into heart disease. Although ultimately these proved disappointing as a stroke treatment, they did signal the beginning of the idea that stroke was a treatable illness. Further progress was made with the development of methods of measuring blood flow in the brain, which led to a greater interest in what happens in the brain during a stroke and how it may recover. Although at this time neurologists were dealing with only 1 to 2 per cent of stroke cases, they led this research. Another step forward came with the recognition that transient ischaemic attacks (TIAs or mini-strokes) could herald a full-blown stroke.

Parallel to the development of more effective medical treatments was the introduction of structured rehabilitation, an important part of stroke care today. Initially led by geriatricians with a team of nurses, physiotherapists and occupational therapists and social workers, this is now recognised as a key aspect of contemporary stroke care. A big step forward came in the 1980s with the introduction of speech therapists to deal with the speech and language problems (dysphasia) that affect many stroke patients.

Today, new insights are arising from the development of more specialised imaging techniques such as magnetic resonance imaging (MRI) and computerised tomography (CT), which can show in detail exactly what is happening in the brain during a stroke.

Initial treatments

If you have a stroke you should be admitted to hospital without delay and see a stroke specialist within 24 hours. It really does make a difference to get there quickly (see Rudd, p.197). If the doctor thinks you have had a stroke he or she should carry out a detailed examination and blood tests to confirm this suspicion. This should involve a CT scan and other tests such as ultrasound of the carotid arteries or, in some centres, an MRI scan, which can look at brain damage in more detail, as well as show the blood vessels supplying the brain (see Markus, p.192; Rudd, p.198).

In the immediate aftermath of a stroke the emphasis will be on keeping you stable, preventing the stroke from progressing and further damage or complications arising (see Tallis, p.200). This will include maintaining the correct balance of fluid and electrolytes (mineral salts) in your blood, preventing your blood pressure from falling to dangerously low levels (hypotension) and minimising the risk of complications such as swelling (oedema) of the brain, heart problems, blood vessel problems and problems affecting the muscles. Further possible complications include seizures, depression, pneumonia, urinary tract infections, muscle contractures and pressure sores caused by lying immobile. You may need to be admitted to intensive care in order for basic functions of life to be supported.

After this initial period the doctor may prescribe a number of different treatments and interventions designed to help your recovery and to prevent you having a further stroke.

Drug treatments

There are many medications that may be prescribed for treating the medical problems arising from a stroke. The precise ones used will depend on what type of stroke you have had and its underlying causes. Common medications used include:

Blood pressure-lowering drugs (antihypertensives)

High blood pressure is the single most important risk factor for stroke. Usually, you won't be prescribed blood pressure-lowering drugs in the first few days following your stroke, as it's possible that a higher blood pressure can actually help maintain better blood flow to the brain. However, if your blood pressure remains high after two to three weeks you may need blood pressure-lowering drugs. There are many different types, all of which act in different ways and can have different side-effects. The doctor will select one or more drugs, although it may require a little trial and error before you find what suits you.

Antiplatelet therapy

Drugs that inhibit the action of platelets (blood cells involved in the process of clotting) can reduce the tendency of blood to clot and prevent a further stroke in some people who have had ischaemic strokes. Perhaps the best-known antiplatelet drug is aspirin. A number of research studies have shown that taking a mini-aspirin (a dose of 50 mg to 325 mg a day) helps reduce the risk of having another stroke. If you are not a suitable candidate for aspirin the doctor may prescribe a different kind of antiplatelet drug. Antiplatelet therapy is not used for haemorrhagic stroke as it can actually worsen the condition.

Anticoagulant therapy

Anticoagulants are another type of medication that interfere with clotting. Probably the most well known is warfarin. Warfarin is a powerful treatment that needs to be very exactly prescribed: too much and there is a risk of haemorrhage; too little and the risk of stroke is increased. For this reason, the doctor will need to do blood tests to measure the speed at which your blood is clotting. Warfarin use is particularly beneficial for patients who had a stroke caused by blood clots coming from the heart. This is most often due to atrial fibrillation (an irregular heartbeat).

Surgery

Sometimes surgery may be needed to remove blood from brain tissues following a haemorrhagic stroke or to correct an underlying weakness in the blood vessels (aneurysm).

Another operation designed to help clear blocked arteries is known as a carotid endarterectomy (see Markus, p.192; Naylor, p.194). If you have had a stroke or TIA, the specialist should do an ultrasound scan to see whether your carotid arteries are blocked and if so how severely. Research suggests that because there is a risk of suffering a stroke during the operation, the balance of risk versus outcome is better in those with greatly blocked arteries. It is best if this operation can be carried out within an integrated service, where the surgeon is operating closely with the stroke specialists (see Markus, p.192) and vital that you ask what your surgeon's rates for complications are.

Rehabilitation

One of the most important features of stroke treatment is rehabilitation. This is designed to help you to:

- regain functions that may have been lost as a result of your stroke

- learn ways of dealing with problems caused by lost abilities
- learn how to manage speech and language problems caused by a stroke
- learn how to manage the activities of daily life, such as dressing or using public transport, that may have been affected by a stroke
- deal with the social, emotional, financial and other consequences of having a stroke.

Currently, rehabilitation services tend to be rather patchy, depending on where you live and the priorities and resources available in your area. For example, you may receive rehabilitation at home, in an outpatient department or day hospital, and services may be provided by a community care team, a general rehabilitation team or a multi-disciplinary stroke rehabilitation team. To be most effective, rehabilitation should begin as soon as possible after you have had a stroke (see Tallis, p.200).

How does that measure up to treatment in the rest of Europe and the USA?

Although medical and surgical treatments are broadly similar, the way stroke care is organised in the rest of Europe differs significantly from treatment in the UK. Recent studies suggest that death rates after a stroke are higher in the UK compared with other European countries such as France and Germany. This may be because in other countries people are more likely to be treated by a neurologist than by a geriatrician. And in the UK there is no age cut-off point for treatment, meaning that statistics will show a higher death rate.

In the USA someone having a stroke will virtually always be admitted to a hospital. Care will tend to be led by a specialist neurologist rather than a geriatrician or general physician, as in the UK. There is much greater use of early, active treatment with clot-busting drugs (thrombolysis) than there is in the UK.

What new treatments are available?

The biggest change has been the introduction in the late 1990s of the use of clot-busting drugs (thrombolytic agents) at an early stage for people who have had ischaemic strokes, to dissolve blood clots blocking blood flow to the brain. This has now been proved to be of value in reducing the amount of brain damage sustained in a stroke.

The treatment tissue plasminogen activator (tPA) has been used to dissolve clots in heart disease for many years and is widely used in the USA. Although the clot busters are a welcome addition, they are suitable only for a small number of patients – moreover, only patients that are already being treated in some form of well-organised stroke care. They need to be rushed in and scanned within three to six hours of suffering a stroke.

Other new approaches include a more aggressive use of blood pressure-lowering drugs such as ACE inhibitors to help prevent subsequent strokes and the use of statins (cholesterol-lowering drugs), designed to help treat and prevent furring of the arteries.

Despite the value of clot-busting drugs, the most effective treatment for stroke patients remains being treated in a stroke unit, which will reduce your chance of death and disability by 20 per cent (see Naylor, p.196; Rudd, p.197). This kind of good, basic care is what saves lives. Unfortunately, a recent audit of stroke care carried out by the Royal College of Physicians (RCP) revealed that just 27 per cent of stroke patients spent most of their hospital stay in a dedicated unit, and only around one-third spent any time at all in one.

Can I get these on the NHS?

Both ACE inhibitors and statins are already widely used for the treatment and prevention of heart disease. Clot-busting treatment (thrombolysis) has until recently been used only in a couple of centres routinely and in a handful more in clinical trials. However, the treatment has now been given a licence by the Medicines Control Agency (MCA) for use in carefully selected patients, and should become more widely available over the next few years.

What treatments are in the pipeline?

A large amount of research is under way to try to discover neuroprotective drugs that will help avoid additional damage to the brain caused by chemicals released by dying brain cells. Several neuroprotective agents are undergoing clinical trials at the moment. One of the most potentially exciting is magnesium salts, which have been shown in animal models to help protect the blood vessels. The Medical Research Council is funding a large, multi-centre trial (IMAGES) designed to test the efficiency of magnesium sulphate if given within 12 hours of the onset of a stroke. Other neuroprotective agents are being evaluated in the USA and elsewhere.

Research is also being carried out into several new surgical techniques, particularly for people who have aneurysms and other problems with their blood vessels that were once considered untreatable. These include revascularisation techniques similar to the bypass operations used for heart patients, which involve grafting another blood vessel to a cerebral artery in order to provide a new channel for blood to reach the brain.

The leading doctors profiled in this chapter have research interests that include: the role played by narrowed carotid arteries in causing a stroke; whether stroke has a genetic component; the possibilities of repairing neurological impairments.

Who treats it?

Some people who have strokes are treated at home by their GP. However, over 70 per cent of people are admitted to hospital to be treated by a general physician, geriatrician or neurologist, together with a multi-disciplinary team of other medical professionals (see Warlow, p.201). A new sub-specialty of stroke medicine is being introduced, which will qualify doctors to register as stroke physicians.

What training will the specialist have?

Before becoming a consultant, your doctor will have had a general medical training, which includes five years at university followed by one year as a House Officer, before gaining registration with the General Medical Council. They will then have spent two to three years as a Senior House Officer in various medical disciplines. This is followed by a five- or six-year period of specialist registrar training in medicine for the elderly or neurology, working in different hospitals, leading to a Certificate of Completion of Specialist Training that is recognised throughout Europe. In the fifth year and post-certification, doctors are encouraged to train to become sub-specialists. Under the new sub-specialty of stroke medicine, doctors are required to do a year's postgraduate training in a specialised stroke unit following their registration. There are currently only a handful of doctors who have undergone this training and a couple of posts in Scotland, although more will come on board in years to come (see Warlow, p.202).

Where will I receive care?

In a variety of different places, which may include a specialist stroke unit at the hospital, in a general, geriatric or neurological ward, in a specialist outpatient clinic at the hospital, or occasionally at an outreach clinic in the community.

What questions should I or my carer ask about treatment?

- Will a CT scan be performed and, if so, when?
- Will an MRI scan be performed and, if so, when?
- What other tests will be performed?
- What kind of stroke has been sustained and what is the extent of damage?
- What is the likelihood of sustaining another stroke?
- Will thrombolysis be performed?
- What other medications will be prescribed?
- How often will medication have to be taken?
- What side-effects can be expected?
- Are there any alternative medications that may be prescribed?
- Are there any clinical trials being performed that I (the person who has had the stroke) can enter?
- Will an operation be performed?

Prevention and lifestyle

- What drugs (e.g. aspirin, cholesterol-lowering drugs (statins), ACE inhibitors) might be prescribed to help prevent a further stroke?
- What lifestyle measures (e.g. diet, exercise, stopping smoking) can be taken to help prevent another stroke?
- Are there any vitamin supplements that may help prevent a further stroke?

Rehabilitation

- How much recovery can reasonably be expected?
- What help is available to aid recovery?
- Is there a specialist rehabilitation team in the area?
- Where will rehabilitation be given – in hospital, in the community, at home?
- Is there a specialist daycare service in the area?
- What help is there for dysphasia (speech and language difficulties)?

- Will I (the person who has had the stroke) have access to a speech therapist?
- Is there a dysphasia support group in the area?
- Will I (the person who has had the stroke) be referred to a physiotherapist?
- Will I (the person who has had the stroke) get to see a psychologist?
- Will I (the person who has had the stroke) have access to an occupational therapist?
- What aids and equipment are available to help with the activities of everyday life?
- How can I (we) find out what aids and equipment are available?
- Which of these are available on the NHS?
- Are there any benefits I (the person who has had the stroke) may be eligible for?
- How do I (we) apply for these?

What will treatment involve?

What your treatment will involve will depend on the type of stroke you had, its severity and where you live. Although things are beginning to change, treatment patterns for stroke are fragmented and inconsistent and may take place in hospital, in the community, at home or in a mixture of the three.

Ideally, your local stroke service should have a specialised stroke unit. However, even if it does you won't always be cared for there. In fact, according to an audit carried out by the Royal College of Physicians, in 2001 only 27 per cent of people who had sustained a stroke spent most of their hospital stay in a stroke unit and only 36 per cent of people spent any time at all in a stroke unit, despite the fact that research shows people fare better if cared for in a dedicated unit.

Immediately following a stroke you should be cared for either in a stroke unit or dedicated stroke ward, or in a unit or ward that also cares for people with other conditions but that is organised to meet the needs of people who have had a stroke. If you aren't admitted to hospital, you should be given information about what emergency services are available and who to contact and how if your condition worsens.

Depending on the area of the brain affected by your stroke, you may sustain mild to severe physical and/or mental damage. Common consequences of a stroke include one-sided paralysis (hemiparesis), problems swallowing and eating (dysphagia), speech and language difficulties (dysphasia), learning difficulties, incontinence, memory loss, behavioural and emotional changes and loss of physical skills such as walking.

Rehabilitation can help you regain abilities you have lost or find new ways of coping with disabilities and with daily activities such as dressing, cooking, shopping, work and leisure. You should also receive social, emotional and practical support to help you. Rehabilitation may involve staying in hospital, being transferred to a different hospital or unit specialising in rehabilitation or being discharged home with rehabilitation provided on an outpatient basis at the hospital stroke unit or a daycare unit in the community or at home. The exact rehabilitation you need will depend on how your stroke has affected you, but may include speech, occupational therapy and/or physiotherapy and help from a psychologist or psychiatrist if you continue to have emotional problems such as depression or anxiety, which is very common and often responds well to treatment.

Treatment will also involve controlling risk factors with drugs or lifestyle changes to try to prevent a subsequent stroke (see above).

If you were employed at the time of your stroke, you may have to stop work for a period or altogether, depending on how severe your stroke was and how badly you were affected.

What is the difference between a well-run and a badly run stroke service?

The Government's National Service Framework for Older People includes a section on stroke, which specifies the four main components of an integrated stroke service. These include:

- **Prevention.** The service should provide ways of identifying, treating and following up people at risk of stroke
- **Immediate care.** This includes care from a specialist stroke team (see p.187)
- **early and continuing rehabilitation**
- **long-term support** For people who have had strokes and their carers.

Based on these, aspects of a well-run stroke service include:

- **Rapid access clinics.** For people who have had mini-strokes (TIAs) to track down and treat any underlying causes such as high blood pressure, high cholesterol, obesity, smoking (see Warlow, p.202)
- **Dedicated stroke wards/beds.** To care for people in the immediate aftermath of their stroke
- **Early CT scanning (within 48 hours).** This is to determine the nature and cause of the stroke
- **Early use of clot-busting drugs where appropriate.**
- **Early tests of function.** For example, a swallowing assessment (see Rudd, p.198), visual assessment and weighing
- **Effective simple drug treatment.** For example, aspirin.
- **Focused rehabilitation services.** These should be either in a dedicated stroke rehabilitation unit, a clinic or through daycare services in the community
- **Information and support.** Also, the involvement of patient support groups such as the Stroke Association.

What makes a REAL difference to getting better?

Research shows that organised stroke care within a specialist stroke unit decreases the risk of death and disability and increases the chances of rehabilitation.

Dedicated stroke unit

A huge amount of research proves that being treated in a dedicated unit with a multi-disciplinary team of specialists who are both knowledgeable about how to care for people who have had strokes and experienced in providing such care is absolutely essential. For every 100 patients managed in such a unit, an extra three will survive.

Multi-disciplinary team

The staff of a stroke unit should include doctors, nurses, physiotherapists, occupational therapists, speech and language therapists and social workers at the very least. Depression is very common following a stroke, so ideally there should be access to psychologists who can help with the emotional consequences.

Early assessment

Research suggests that an early assessment of the type of stroke and the extent of brain damage is crucial. There should be greater availability of CT and MRI scanners.

Individually tailored care

The precise treatments you need will depend on what type of stroke you had and how severe it was. However, a number of procedures have been shown to be particularly important in trials. These include measures to prevent you developing a blood clot (deep vein thrombosis), the early use of antibiotics for suspected infections, and keeping an eye on your nutritional needs. Getting you moving as quickly as possible to prevent complications caused by prolonged immobility is also important.

Medical management of risk factors

A number of large research studies have shown that medical and surgical treatments can substantially reduce the incidence of a second or future stroke. These include:

- controlling high blood pressure
- using aspirin to keep the blood flowing smoothly and avoid the development of clots following a TIA
- carotid endarterectomy
- stopping smoking
- using warfarin in people with a particular kind of irregular heart rhythm called atrial fibrillation.

Will I get better treatment if I go privately?

There's no evidence that private treatment is better for stroke, as many of the interventions are a matter not of cost but of the availability of an organised stroke service (see Markus, p.191). If you do decide to go privately, you should see a stroke specialist and ideally be looked after by a specialised stroke team.

Will I get better treatment if I go abroad?

It would be difficult for people who have had strokes to travel abroad in the crucial early days following a stroke. Some of the new operations that are being researched for the treatment of certain kinds of stroke may be more available in the USA. However, many of them are still experimental, are likely to be very expensive and may not be suitable for everyone. You also have to take into account the cost of travelling and staying abroad, as well as being away from the support of family and friends.

What support will I be offered by the hospital and are there any independent support groups I can join?

The hospital should provide you with full written information in a form you can understand about your stroke and how it will be treated, as well as information about rehabilitation and any specific problems such as dysphasia, depression or incontinence. In many areas, the hospital will be able to put you in touch with the Stroke Association's community services, which include dysphasia and family support services. Over 400 stroke clubs are also affiliated to the Association, where people who have had strokes can meet and share their experiences.

Useful addresses

Different Strokes
9 Canon Harnett Court
Wolverton Mill
Milton Keynes MK12 5NF
Tel 0845 130 7172
Email: info@differentstrokes.co.uk
www.differentstrokes.co.uk

The Stroke Association
Whitecross Street
London EC1Y 8JJ
Tel 020 7566 0300
National Stroke Helpline 0845 30 33 100
www.stroke.org.uk

Expert opinions

Professor Hugh Markus

People who have suffered a mini-stroke, or transient ischaemic attack (TIA), should get to a dedicated TIA clinic within a week, even if it means travelling to another district. But in this situation you are better off getting to an NHS clinic than paying to go private, says Hugh Markus, Professor of Neurology at St George's Hospital in London.

'If you have had a TIA, you really need to see someone who is running a TIA service rather than be seen in a general neurology or medical clinic,' he says. 'Quite often people go privately to a general neurologist, but I think you shouldn't see a generalist, you should see someone who is doing it all the time. Not every district will have a rapid access service, but certainly with TIAs you can be referred across districts because you are mobile.'

Having a TIA is a major indicator that a person is in danger of having a stroke. And as well as medical expertise, a dedicated TIA clinic has access to a range of other services aimed at helping people to control this risk. 'In our clinic, we have a stroke prevention nurse who will counsel all patients on how to reduce the risk of stroke. The nurse is also able to give them lifestyle advice on coping with stroke: how it affects driving, occupation, sex and other issues.'

Many patients visiting TIA clinics have a narrowing in the carotid artery, a major blood vessel in the neck. The deposits or plaques in this artery are implicated in the formation of blood clots that can go on to cause strokes and TIAs, so appropriate assessment and integrated treatment of this condition are vital components of a good TIA service.

Two imaging technologies are used to assess narrowing of the carotid arteries, and it is important that those at risk are referred for a scan. The most common technique is called duplex scanning, and involves using ultrasound to look at the degree of carotid narrowing. But a newer alternative, called MR-angiography, is available at some centres, and this can give an almost complete picture of blood flow within the brain.

Those with severe stenosis (narrowing) should be seen by a vascular surgeon so that they can be considered for an operation called carotid endarterectomy, in which the carotid plaques are removed. However, Markus feels that it is important that the surgeon is operating closely with stroke specialists, and not in isolation. 'If you are going on to have carotid endarterectomy, you need to make sure that it is done within an integrated service. You don't want to be referred to a surgeon; you want to be referred to a service with a stroke doctor who will interact with the surgeons. For example, we meet every two weeks with the surgeon and the radiologist to discuss all of our patients with narrowing of the carotid artery, so we have integrated management.'

Improving the understanding of the role played by narrowed carotid arteries in causing stroke is an important research objective for Markus. He is currently using both ultrasound and magnetic resonance (MR) scanning to study the tiny blood clots, or emboli, that are produced by the diseased blood vessels.

'These emboli appear to predict stroke in people with narrowed carotid arteries, and we are looking at ways to switch them off with therapy,' he says. 'One way is to see whether we can actually predict stroke risk and use it to select patients for surgery. We're doing a large multi-centre study to see if this is possible. The second way is by assessing novel drug therapies. Because these emboli are much more common than stroke itself, we can study far smaller groups of patients and still have enough statistical power to tell if one treatment is better than another.'

Some people who have strokes do not have conventional risk factors, and Markus is also looking at whether stroke has a genetic component. The fact that there are differences in both the type and frequency of strokes in people from ethnic minority groups adds weight to the idea that genes are involved. Markus is studying this effect in the minority communities of south London. 'We are particularly interested in stroke in people of African-Caribbean ethnicity, because they have about double the risk,' he says. 'They also tend to get stroke about ten years earlier and have a different distribution of types of stroke.'

If the genes responsible can be identified and their role in causing stroke ascertained, Markus hopes that the door will be opened on new therapies for treating and preventing the condition in the future. At the moment, though, his advice for people who are at risk from a stroke is to get to a specialist clinic as fast as possible, even if it means looking outside the local area.

Mr Ross Naylor

There are wide variations in outcomes between UK units performing a common operation on the carotid artery in the neck. The operation, carotid endarterectomy, can significantly reduce the chance that the patient will go on to suffer a stroke, and a large number of units now perform it. However, the number of cases seen by individual surgeons varies widely, and Mr Ross Naylor, a consultant vascular surgeon at Leicester Royal Infirmary, believes it vital that patients ask their surgeon about their own risk before consenting to the procedure.

About 80 per cent of strokes are caused by blockage of an artery inside the brain. In up to half of these, the patient will have previously developed a narrowing (stenosis) of the carotid artery. The carotid arteries are the main blood supply to the brain and lie on either side of the neck. A blood clot (thrombus) forms on the surface of the stenoses and can break off and pass into the brain circulation (embolism). Depending on the size of the blood clot, the patient may suffer a mini-stroke or transient ischaemic attack (TIA), while larger emboli will cause disabling strokes. Carotid endarterectomy aims to remove the stenosis before a major stroke occurs. Although its long-term effectiveness has been proven in large clinical trials around the world, the operation itself can cause death or stroke in a small number of patients.

'In the late 1980s and early 1990s, carotid surgery tended to be concentrated at the bigger centres. There has been a trend since towards a proliferation of centres doing carotid surgery, which has matched the proliferation of vascular units across the country. And there is a debate within the vascular and stroke professional associations as to whether it would be better to go back to doing larger numbers of procedures in fewer centres, so as to concentrate the experience.'

'The operative mortality rate is about 1 per cent,' says Naylor. 'In our unit, the 30-day risk of death and/or stroke (the operative risk) has been 2.6 per cent following the last 850 operations, but that can vary quite extensively around the country. It could be as high as 7 or 8 per cent in some centres. The key thing you must know is what your surgeon's risks are – I cannot overstate that.'

The vascular unit at Leicester Royal Infirmary set up a carotid surgery research programme in 1992, and over the last ten years there has been a significant reduction in the risks associated with the procedure. 'We found that 6 per cent of patients died or had a stroke within 30 days of surgery,' he says. 'Of those six, four would wake up with a stroke (an intra-operative stroke). The research programme showed that the commonest reason for this type of stroke was the accumulation of small amounts of blood clot on the inner lining of the "cleaned" artery towards the end of the operation. Those thrombi then embolised to the brain causing a stroke. Now we use a tiny camera to have a look at the lining of the artery. If we find any clots, we can remove them before they embolise. By doing this, the six vascular surgeons at the Infirmary and the Leicester General have reduced the risk of intra-operative stroke from 4 per cent to 0.2 per cent following the last 1,200 operations.'

Research went on to show that the main cause of post-operative stroke (after recovery from anaesthesia) was the gradual accumulation of blood clots on the lining of the artery that had just been cleared out. These clots could either embolise into the brain or become so large that they blocked off the carotid artery. The Leicester unit used transcranial Doppler ultrasound to identify patients at high risk of progressing on to a post-operative thrombotic stroke. This machine can actually identify the tiny emboli entering the brain circulation. Special drugs were then given to prevent strokes from progressing. 'This second protocol has transformed our practice,' says Naylor. 'Since we introduced post-operative transcranial Doppler monitoring in 1995, we have done over 850 operations and we have not encountered one stroke due to post-operative carotid thrombosis.'

Despite these advances, carotid endarterectomy can never be wholly risk free, even at a unit like Leicester that specialises in the procedure. Deciding whether or not to operate on a person with narrowed carotid arteries can be tricky for both surgeon and patient, as this is one of very few operations that can be termed 'prophylactic': it is aimed solely at preventing a problem from occurring in the future. 'If you have cancer of the rectum and you don't have an operation, you will develop disseminated cancer. But if you have a transient ischaemic attack [TIA] and a severe carotid stenosis and you don't have an operation, there is still a 75 per cent chance that you will be stroke free at three years.'

The 75 per cent chance of remaining stroke free can be increased to around 90 per cent with surgery, so it is important that people who are high-risk consult a vascular surgeon promptly. At the moment, rapid investigation and intervention can be a bit of a lottery. 'Patients take pot-luck really as to whether there is an established cerebrovascular clinic in their area that can serve them within a short period of time,' says Naylor. 'Put it this way, if it was my dad and he had a TIA, I would want him seen as fast as possible, because the risks of stroke are highest within the first four weeks of having the first mini-stroke.'

'There is increasing evidence that TIA patients should be fast-tracked through the system. But a nationwide consistent emphasis on primary and secondary prevention is just not there for stroke patients. They often feel overwhelmed, neglected and unsupported.'

Whether they get there quickly or not, Naylor's message to patients considering carotid surgery is that they must ask the surgeon who will be performing the operation what their own rates for complications are. Because rates vary so widely, this information is vital for attaining an accurate idea of the risks involved.

Dr Tony Rudd

Stroke care in the UK is still not good enough, says Dr Tony Rudd, the lead stroke physician at St Thomas' Hospital in London. But stroke patients or their relatives can take steps to raise the standard of their own care and drive improvements to the service as a whole. Rudd chairs the Intercollegiate Stroke Working Party, a body that is responsible for drawing up the national clinical guidelines for treating stroke and monitoring their implementation across the NHS.

When someone suffers a stroke, their ability to communicate may be compromised, and it falls to the people around them to take the steps necessary to ensure that they get the best possible care. A critical first step is to get to hospital quickly. 'When someone has a stroke at home,' says Rudd, 'forget about GPs, forget about any other community services, call the ambulance and come straight to hospital. It really does make a difference to get to hospital quickly, as this is not a disease that can be effectively managed in the community.'

Once at the hospital, stroke patients fare best in a dedicated stroke unit. 'Admission to a stroke unit is possibly the single most important factor in improving outcomes for stroke patients,' says Rudd. 'There is plenty of evidence to suggest that the number of people who die following stroke can be reduced by 20 per cent if they are treated in a stroke unit staffed by doctors and nurses with specialist training in the area. That is a huge difference; certainly more than any single drug used to treat stroke.'

At present, however, only a lucky few patients are admitted to one of these units. A recent audit of stroke care carried out by the Royal College of Physicians (RCP) revealed that just 27 per cent of stroke patients spent most of their hospital stay in a dedicated unit, and only around one-third spent any time at all in one. In 1999, this figure was 25 per cent, so at the current rate of change it would take over 70 years before all patients admitted to hospital with strokes spend half their time in a stroke unit.

Whether they are admitted to a stroke unit or not, Rudd believes that all stroke patients should expect to be seen by a specialist doctor early during their stay. 'The hospital may only have one consultant who specialises in stroke, so it is not always possible to be seen straightaway,' he says. 'But you ought to be referred to a stroke specialist within 24 hours of being admitted.'

As well as seeing a specialist, patients need to have a brain scan before steps can be taken to protect the brain from further damage. This critically important scan, which is used to distinguish between strokes that have been caused by a blood clot (infarction) and those caused by a haemorrhage, is sometimes not performed early enough or may be missed altogether. Knowing the type of stroke is crucial for doctors, as drugs that can benefit patients with blood clots can have adverse effects on those with haemorrhages and vice versa.

The RCP audit revealed that at present nearly one in five stroke patients is not given a brain scan, and Rudd's advice is to be persistent. 'A brain scan is the only way to tell an infarction from a haemorrhage, and anyone who tells you otherwise doesn't know what they are talking about,' he says.

It is also important to have a swallowing assessment performed early, as the swallowing reflex may have been damaged by the stroke. Stroke patients staying on general wards, where staff have not necessarily had specialist training, are sometimes offered food or drink which they are unable to swallow properly, contributing to the risk of a damaging chest infection. This is another area where it pays to be vigilant. 'If the patient is being offered a cup of tea,' says Rudd, 'it's worth checking with the nurses that they have had a swallowing assessment and it is okay for them.'

Rudd's knowledge of the pitfalls of non-specialist stroke care comes from personal experience. He was appointed as a consultant geriatrician and general physician at St Thomas' in 1988, before the hospital opened a stroke unit. 'We made a decision as a department that stroke care within the hospital was pretty abysmal. Patients were all being managed by general physicians on lots of different wards. One of the first things we did was to establish a rehabilitation stroke unit using a ward previously providing geriatric rehabilitation, aiming to bring patients with complex problems to the unit as soon as possible after admission,' he says. 'Different hospitals have different ways of managing stroke, and there is no absolute right or wrong way. The important thing is that you get seen by somebody who knows about stroke fairly quickly after being admitted.'

Professor Raymond Tallis

Only a small proportion of the people at risk of having a stroke receive effective preventive therapies, according to Raymond Tallis, Professor of Geriatric Medicine at the University of Manchester. With chronic under-provision in UK stroke services and an ever-increasing number of people suffering strokes, he believes that improved strategies for preventing strokes will be the most important factor in modernising stroke care in the NHS. 'All the real gains are going to be in identifying the risk factors and treating them,' he says. 'That will make a massive difference.'

Stroke risk factors, such as a prior history of strokes, smoking or high blood pressure (hypertension), are not being effectively treated in primary care. But raising awareness among GPs and compliance among their patients could lead to a dramatic reduction in the number of stroke emergencies. 'Just to give you one example, half the people with hypertension are still not diagnosed. Half of those who are diagnosed don't get treated. Half of those who get treated still don't reach the target levels. There is a huge slack to take up in prevention, so if you want to get the best out of the system, prevention is the first thing,' he says.

Stroke is the single largest cause of disability in the UK, and Tallis's research and clinical work is focused on the rehabilitation of stroke sufferers. In particular, he is looking at ways to encourage the brain to recover from the damage caused by stroke. 'Chronic neurological disability is the single biggest challenge now facing the health service, and there is plenty of evidence that with new strategies and approaches we will be able to deliver something useful to patients,' he says. 'The existing therapies have been very good at helping patients to adapt to impairment and helping to remove barriers to recovery. What we've been not so good at is driving recovery from damage. Our own research over the last 20 years has been looking at what the recovering nervous system actually needs: what kind of inputs would actually drive recovery.'

It is information from basic science that is providing the answers. Laboratory work using animals and new imaging techniques that show how the brain functions have revealed that it is capable of rewiring and reorganising itself to minimise the effects of damage. It is hoped that methods such as electrical stimulation and tailored exercises will be able to encourage the process.

Neurological repair is an exciting new avenue in stroke therapy, but it is still in its infancy. There are, however, simple steps that a stroke service can take to protect a patient's brain from unnecessary damage in the critical early stages of treatment.

'The important thing is that you are in a set-up that is completely geared up to making sure that there is secondary prevention, so you don't have a further stroke,' says Tallis. 'It's also very important that the service looks after your brain in the acute phase, making sure that it is oxygenated and that there is enough fluid. Then there is a need to make sure you have reasonably intense, prompt, appropriate, intelligent, multi-disciplinary rehabilitation. There is plenty of evidence now that if you go into that sort of set-up rather than the general hurly-burly, your chances of being dead or disabled after six months are reduced by over 30 per cent, which completely dwarfs any benefits from drugs.'

While stroke has an acute onset, it has a lifetime's consequences, and the interface between acute stroke services and long-term rehabilitation can be a problem area, with patients feeling they have been abandoned once they leave the hospital. 'It is very important when you've had a stroke that there is a system keeping an eye on you, so if new things happen or you go into a spiral of shrinkage of life-space because you are giving up, people will pick it up and report you. There should be an agreed point of contact,' says Tallis.

Despite the widely reported under-investment in stroke services, the new trends in rehabilitation aimed at repairing neurological impairments offer a source of hope to those who have suffered a stroke. However, a well-organised stroke service should already be taking active steps to reduce neurological damage in the immediate aftermath of stroke, and much more can be done to prevent strokes from occurring in the first place.

Professor Charles Warlow

Despite the fact that stroke is a brain disorder, traditionally it has not been treated by neurologists in the UK. Instead, a number of medical specialties, of which the most important is geriatrics, have taken shared responsibility for the treatment of stroke patients.

Poor integration between the different specialties, together with lack of funding, have seen stroke services suffer. But the emergence of a new specialty – stroke medicine – may help to alleviate these difficulties, says Professor Charles Warlow, an expert in stroke who works at the Western General Hospital in Edinburgh.

As President of the Association of British Neurologists, Warlow knows only too well of the historical attitude of his own specialty to stroke patients. 'Neurologists generally have been uninterested in stroke in the UK. Not so in Europe, nor in America. But traditionally in the UK neurologists have turned their backs on stroke,' he says. 'This is partly because there have been very few of us and partly because of a sort of elitism: we don't do stroke.'

Traditionally, stroke patients were left to languish on general wards under the care of doctors who lacked specialist training in the condition. And when specialist stroke units did begin to emerge, it was geriatricians who assumed responsibility for running them. Whatever the specialty, however, Warlow points out that the most important thing is to see a doctor who is interested in the condition.

'When you ask where you would go with a stroke, you would want to go somewhere with a well-organised stroke service run by somebody who was knowledgeable and enthusiastic about stroke. That person is more likely to be a geriatrician than a neurologist, but it could be either,' he says.

There are circumstances where patients admitted with strokes can benefit from seeing a neurologist. These include cases where the diagnosis is unclear, there are unexpected symptoms or the patient is not from a typical risk group. Most hospitals do not have neurologists available all the time, and this has led to friction between the specialties.

'There are some geriatricians who would regard neurologists as completely useless because they only turn up a week late and don't contribute anything – and sometimes they have a point,' says Warlow. 'But one would like to think that the skills of a trained neurologist and a trained geriatrician can be brought together to provide a really good stroke service, which can call on all the skills that are required without these dreadful turf wars.'

A solution to this problem is emerging in the form of a new specialty dedicated to treating stroke, which will encompass the relevant parts of geriatrics, neurology, clinical pharmacology and rehabilitation. The British Association of Stroke Physicians, which includes representatives from all these specialties, is the driving force behind this change. 'There is now a training programme that has been recognised by the Royal College of Physicians, and there is a sub-committee that oversees training. But this is still very early days,' he says.

Certainly, the new doctors will face formidable problems, not least with prompt access to other essential facilities like computerised tomography (CT) scanners, which are important in determining the type of stroke a person has suffered. 'Every service has got a scanner, but they don't always use it,' says Warlow. 'Some close up at four o'clock on Friday afternoon and reopen on Monday at nine. It's getting better, but it's not just a shortage in neurology; it's a shortage of everything in the NHS.'

Shortages elsewhere can have a detrimental impact on even the best initiatives in stroke care. An example of this can be seen in rapid access neurovascular or TIA clinics, which are designed to provide people who have had mini-strokes with prompt access to specialists.

'The slight downside to these clinics is that 50 per cent of the patients we see in our rapid access clinic don't have strokes or TIAs at all – they've got brain tumours, migraine and epilepsy,' says Warlow. 'These are important problems that need sorting out, but the average neurologist's routine waiting time is something like six months, and of course GPs will try to get round that by saying, "Ah, a rapid access neurovascular clinic!"'

Despite these problems, Warlow believes that stroke services have improved greatly in the last ten years, and for the future, we can expect specialist stroke consultants coming through a tailored training programme to continue the trend.

Specialist directory

How to use the directory

This directory is meant to give you an idea of the leading specialists in the UK in the areas covered by the book. Our website (www.drfoster.co.uk) gives more information about consultants and different specialties.

It is important to remember that this information should be used in conjunction with your GP. UK consultants usually only accept patients who have been referred to them by another doctor, normally a GP. Furthermore, GPs often have a good idea of the strengths and weakness of consultants working in their local hospitals, which form the basis of their recommendations.

We have listed consultants who we found in our analysis to have produced a large amount of high quality clinical research into these areas. The analysis was carried out on our behalf by City University. The consultants who are named have demonstrated that they know a great deal about the clinical area in which they have done research. It should be remembered, however, that this is not necessarily the same as showing a high degree of clinical skill. However, in the absence of other information with which to choose a consultant to treat one of these conditions, we consider this to be a good place to start. It should also be noted that we cannot be certain that the analysis will have identified all research papers in the area and there may be consultants who have carried out research that we are unaware of.

Award

This column refers to merit awards, given to consultants for exemplary performance within the NHS. They are judged on a range of criteria, only one of which is professional excellence. This means that, while the consultants receiving merit awards are expected to demonstrate this excellence, it does not necessarily mean that their clinical skills are superior to those of a consultant who does not have a merit award.

Grad.

This indicates the year of a consultant's medical qualification.

Arthritis specialists

Name	Hospital	Award	Grad.
Dr A Bell	Musgrave Park Hospital, Belfast		1976
Prof H Bird	Leeds General Infirmary	A	1970
Dr A Calin	Royal National Hospital for Rheumatic Diseases, Bath		1968
Dr M I Cawley	Salisbury District Hospital	B	1958
Dr J Compston	Addenbrooke's Hospital, Cambridge	B	1970
Prof C Cooper	Southampton General Hospital	B	1980
Dr P J Dawes	Haywood Centre, Stoke on Trent	B	1976
Dr D D'Cruz	St Thomas' Hospital, London		1983
Prof M Doherty	Nottingham City Hospital	B	1975
Dr D Doyle	Whipps Cross University Hospital, London	A	1972
Prof R Eastell	Northern General Hospital, Sheffield		1977
Prof J C Edwards	Middlesex and University College Hospitals, London		1974
Prof P Emery	Leeds General Infirmary		1977
Dr R Francis	Freeman Hospital, Newcastle General Hospital, Royal Victoria Infirmary, Newcastle upon Tyne		1975
Dr K Gaffney	Norfolk and Norwich University Hospital, Norwich		1988
Prof J S Gaston	Addenbrooke's Hospital, Cambridge		1976
Prof D Haskard	Hammersmith Hospital, London	A	1977
Dr B Hazleman	Addenbrooke's Hospital, Cambridge	A	1965
Dr A Herrick	Hope Hospital, Salford		1981
Dr E Ho Choy	King's College Hospital, London		1985
Prof D Hosking	Nottingham City Hospital	A	1966
Dr G R Hughes	St Thomas' Hospital, London	APLUS	1964
Prof D Isenberg	Middlesex and University College Hospitals, London	A	1973
Dr M Khamashta	St Thomas' Hospital, London		1983

Dr G Kingsley	University Hospital Lewisham, London	B	1979
Dr J Kirwan	Bristol Royal Infirmary		1974
Dr A MacGregor	St Thomas' Hospital, London		1984
Prof R Maini	Charing Cross Hospital, London	APLUS	1962
Prof P Mang Woo	Great Ormond Street Hospital for Children, London	A	1972
Dr N McHugh	Royal National Hospital for Rheumatic Diseases, Bath		1978
Prof G Panayi	Guy's Hospital, London	A	1965
Dr C Pitzalis	King's College Hospital, London		1983
S Ralston	Aberdeen Royal Infirmary	B	1978
Prof D Reid	Aberdeen Royal Infirmary		1975
Prof C O Savage	Queen Elizabeth Hospital, Birmingham	B	1978
Prof D G Scott	Norfolk and Norwich University Hospital, Norwich	B	1973
Prof A Silman	Manchester Royal Infirmary	B	1974
Dr T Spector	St Thomas' Hospital, London		1982
Prof R Sturrock	Glasgow Royal Infirmary		1969
Prof D P Symmons	Macclesfield District General Hospital		1977
Dr P J Venables	Charing Cross Hospital, London	B	1972
Prof M Walport	Hammersmith Hospital, London	A	1977
Dr R Watts	Ipswich Hospital		1982
Dr A Woolf	Royal Cornwall Hospital, Truro	B	1975
Dr G Wright	The Royal Hospitals, Belfast		1987

Private patients only:

Prof M I V Jayson	BUPA Hospital Manchester		1961

Asthma specialists

Name	Hospital	Award	Grad.
Prof J Ayres	Birmingham Heartlands Hospital	B	1987
Dr N Barnes	London Chest Hospital		1979
P Barnes	Royal Brompton Hospital, London	APLUS	1972
Dr P Barry	Leicester Royal Infirmary		1984
Dr S Bourke	Royal Victoria Infirmary, Newcastle upon Tyne		1981
Dr P Bradding	Glenfield Hospital, Leicester		1985
Prof J Britton	Nottingham City Hospital		1978
Dr P Burge	Birmingham Heartlands Hospital	A	1969
Dr A Bush	Royal Brompton Hospital, London		1978
Prof P M Calverley	University Hospital Aintree, Liverpool	B	1973
Prof K Chung	Royal Brompton Hospital, London		1975
Dr M Connolly	Manchester Royal Infirmary		1980
Dr C Corrigan	Guy's Hospital, London		1983
Dr J Costello	King's College Hospital, London	A	1968
Snr Lect Med R Djukanovic	Southampton General Hospital		1978
I J Doull	University Hospital of Wales, Cardiff		1984
Prof A Frew	Southampton General Hospital		1980
Prof J A Friend	Aberdeen Royal Infirmary	A	1962
Prof I Hall	Queen's Medical Centre, Nottingham		1982
Dr B D Harrison	Norfolk and Norwich University Hospital, Norwich	A	1967
Dr L Heaney	Belfast City Hospital		1988
Prof P Helms	Royal Aberdeen Children's Hospital		1972
Prof D Hendrick	Royal Victoria Infirmary, Newcastle upon Tyne	B	1966
J Hopkin	Singleton Hospital, Swansea	B	1972
Dr P Howarth	Royal South Hants Hospital, Southampton		1976

Dr P Ind	Hammersmith Hospital, London	B	1974
Prof A Kay	Royal Brompton Hospital, London	APLUS	1963
Dr O Kon	St Mary's Hospital, London		1988
Dr J Legge	Aberdeen Royal Infirmary	B	1966
Prof B Lipworth	Ninewells Hospital, Dundee		1983
Prof A Morice	Castle Hill Hospital, Cottingham		1978
Prof C O'Callaghan	Leicester Royal Infirmary		1982
Dr B O'Connor	King's College Hospital, London		1980
Dr I Pavord	Glenfield Hospital, Leicester		1984
Prof J Price	King's College Hospital, London	A	1969
N Pride	Hammersmith Hospital, London	A	1955
Dr A Redington	Hull Royal Infirmary		1984
Dr C Scadding	Royal National Throat, Nose and Ear Hospital, London	B	1972
Dr K Tan	Wishaw General Hospital		1989
Prof A Tattersfield	Nottingham City Hospital	APLUS	1963
Prof N Thomson	Gartnavel General Hospital, Glasgow		1972
Prof A Wardlaw	Glenfield Hospital, Leicester		1980
Prof J Warner	Southampton General Hospital	A	1968
Prof A Woodcock	Wythenshawe Hospital, Manchester	B	1975

Breast cancer specialists

Name	Hospital	Award	Grad.
Prof T Anderson	Western General Hospital, Edinburgh		1962
Dr B Angus	Royal Victoria Infirmary, Newcastle upon Tyne	B	1975
Mr A Baildam	Withington Hospital, Manchester		1978
Prof R Blamey	Nottingham City Hospital	APLUS	1960
Dr L Bobrow	Addenbrooke's Hospital, Cambridge		1962
Prof N Bundred	Wythenshawe Hospital, Manchester		1980
Dr J Buscombe	Royal Free Hospital, London		1984
Dr D Cameron	Western General Hospital, Edinburgh		1986
Mr R Carpenter	St Bartholomew's Hospital, London		1980
Mr U Chetty	Western General Hospital, Edinburgh		1970
Prof T Cooke	Glasgow Royal Infirmary		1973
Prof R C D Coombes	Charing Cross Hospital, London	A	1971
Mr J Dixon	Western General Hospital, Edinburgh		1978
I Ellis	Nottingham City Hospital	B	1978
Dr P Ellis	Guy's Hospital, London		1986
Prof C Elston	Nottingham City Hospital	A	1961
Prof O Eremin	Lincoln County Hospital	A	1964
Dr A Evans	Nottingham City Hospital		1984
Prof I Fentiman	Guy's Hospital, London	B	1968
Mr J N Fox	Castle Hill Hospital, Cottingham		1972
K Gatter	John Radcliffe Hospital, Headington	B	1979
Regius Prof W George	Western Infirmary, Glasgow		1966
Mr G Gui	Royal Marsden Hospital, London		1986
Prof A Harris	Churchill Hospital, Headington	A	1973
Prof S Heys	Aberdeen Royal Infirmary		1981

Dr A J Hilson	Royal Free Hospital, London	B	1967
Mr K Horgan	Leeds General Infirmary		1979
Dr J Houghton	Countess of Chester Hospital, Chester	B	1965
Dr A Hutcheon	Aberdeen Royal Infirmary		1968
Dr S R Johnston	Royal Marsden Hospital, London		1986
Dr A Jones	Royal Free Hospital, London		1989
Mr M Kissin	Royal Surrey County Hospital, Guildford		1975
A H Lee	Nottingham City Hospital		1985
Prof T W Lennard	Royal Victoria Infirmary, Newcastle upon Tyne	B	1977
Prof R C Leonard	Singleton Hospital, Swansea		1971
Dr B Magee	Christie Hospital, Manchester		1980
Dr A Makris	Mount Vernon Hospital, Northwood		1985
Prof R Mansel	University Hospital of Wales, Cardiff	A	1971
Dr D Miles	Guy's Hospital, London		1981
Prof K Mokbel	St George's Hospital, London		1990
Prof P Mortimer	St George's Hospital, London	B	1975
Dr A Neal	Royal Surrey County Hospital, Guildford		1985
Prof J Carmichael	Nottingham City Hospital	B	1975
Dr S Pinder	Nottingham City Hospital		1986
Prof T Powles	Royal Marsden Hospital, Sutton	A	1964
Mr A Purushotham	Addenbrooke's Hospital, Cambridge		1983
Mr R Rainsbury	Royal Hampshire County Hospital, Winchester	B	1974
Prof A Ramirez	St Thomas' Hospital, London		1982
Dr A Reid	Glasgow Royal Infirmary		1980
Prof J F Robertson	Nottingham City Hospital		1980
Mr G Royle	Southampton General Hospital		1970
Prof R Rubens	Guy's Hospital, London	A	1967
Mr N P Sacks	Royal Marsden Hospital, London		1980
Mr R Sainsbury	Middlesex and University College Hospitals, London	B	1977

Dr T Sarkar	Aberdeen Royal Infirmary	B	1966
Prof D T Sharpe	Bradford Royal Infirmary	A	1970
Mr H Sinnett	Charing Cross Hospital, London		1972
D Smith	Victoria Infirmary, Glasgow	B	1966
Professor I Smith	Royal Marsden Hospital, London	A	1971
Prof C Steel	Western General Hospital, Edinburgh		1965
Prof (Miss) R Walker	Glenfield Hospital, Leicester	A	1971
Dr C Wells	St Bartholomew's Hospital, London		1977
Dr A R Wilson	Nottingham City Hospital	B	1979
Prof J Yarnold	Royal Marsden Hospital, Sutton	B	1972
Mr C Yiangou	Queen Alexandra Hospital, Portsmouth		1987

Colorectal cancer specialists

Name	Hospital	Award	Grad.
Prof T Allen-Mersh	Chelsea and Westminster Hospital, London		1973
Prof R H Begent	Royal Free Hospital, London	A	1967
Prof P Boulos	Middlesex and University College Hospitals, London	B	1966
Prof J Cassidy	Western Infirmary, Glasgow		1981
Dr D Cunningham	Royal Marsden Hospital, London	B	1978
M Dunlop	Western General Hospital, Edinburgh	B	1982
Mr G Duthie	Castle Hill Hospital, Cottingham		1983
Dr D G Evans	Manchester Royal Infirmary		1983
Mr R Farouk	Royal Berkshire and Battle Hospitals, Reading		1986
Mr P Finan	Leeds General Infirmary	B	1974
Prof P Guillou	St James's University Hospital, Leeds	APLUS	1970
Mr N Hall	Addenbrooke's Hospital, Cambridge		1985
Mr M Hershman	Royal Liverpool University Hospital		1980
Dr T F Hickish	Poole Hospital		1984
Dr S Hodgson	Guy's Hospital, London	B	1969
Dr P Johnston	Belfast City Hospital	B	1982
Mr D Kumar	St George's Hospital, London	B	1975
Prof P W Lee	Hull Royal Infirmary	A	1968
Prof C Marks	Royal Surrey County Hospital, Guildford	A	1967
Prof J Monson	Castle Hill Hospital, Cottingham	B	1979
Mr B Moran	North Hampshire Hospital, Basingstoke		1980
Prof N J Mortensen	John Radcliffe Hospital, Headington	B	1973
Prof J M Northover	St Mark's Hospital, Harrow	A	1970
Prof R K Phillips	St Mark's Hospital, Harrow	B	1975

Prof J Primrose	Southampton General Hospital		1977
Mr A Radcliffe	Llandough Hospital, Penarth		1971
Mr M H Robinson	Queen's Medical Centre, Nottingham		1983
Mr P Rooney	Royal Liverpool University Hospital		1984
Prof J Scholefield	Queen's Medical Centre, Nottingham		1983
Prof R J Steele	Ninewells Hospital, Dundee	B	1977
Prof I Taylor	Middlesex and University College Hospitals, London	APLUS	1968
Mr M Thomas	Bristol Royal Infirmary		1984
Dr C Williams	St Mark's Hospital, Harrow		1962
Prof N Williams	Royal London Hospital	APLUS	1970

Diabetes specialists

Name	Hospital	Award	Grad.
Dr C Acerini	Addenbrooke's Hospital, Cambridge		1988
Prof S Amiel	King's College Hospital, London	B	1978
Prof A Atkinson	The Royal Hospitals, Belfast		1973
Prof P Baylis	Royal Victoria Infirmary, Newcastle upon Tyne	APLUS	1970
Dr P Bingley	Southmead Hospital, Bristol		1994
Dr H Bodansky	Leeds General Infirmary, Leeds		1974
Prof A J Boulton	Manchester Royal Infirmary		1976
Dr A Burden	Leicester General Hospital	B	1970
Dr D Cavan	Royal Bournemouth Hospital		1985
Dr T Dornan	Hope Hospital, Salford	B	1975
Prof B Frier	Royal Infirmary of Edinburgh	B	1972
Dr G Gill	John Thompson Day Case Unit, Liverpool	B	1972
Dr R Greenwood	Norfolk and Norwich University Hospital, Norwich	B	1968
Dr A Hattersley	Royal Devon and Exeter Hospital, Exeter		1984
Dr S Heller	Northern General Hospital, Sheffield		1977
Prof G Hitman	Royal London Hospital, London	B	1976
P Home	Freeman Hospital, Newcastle General Hospital, Royal Victoria Infirmary, Newcastle upon Tyne	B	1976
Dr D Humphriss	Scarborough General Hospital		1985
D Johnston	St Mary's Hospital, London	A	1971
Prof R Jung	Ninewells Hospital, Dundee	A	1972
Prof R D Leslie	St Bartholomew's Hospital, London		1972
Dr I Macfarlane	University Hospital Aintree, Liverpool	B	1973
Dr M Mansfield	St James's University Hospital, Leeds		1987
Dr D Matthews	Radcliffe Infirmary, Oxford	B	1975
Dr K Matyka	Birmingham Heartlands Hospital		1984

Dr M Nattrass	Selly Oak Hospital, Birmingham	B	1970
R Newton	Ninewells Hospital, Dundee	APLUS	1969
Prof S O'Rahilly	Addenbrooke's Hospital, Cambridge	B	1981
Dr P Perros	Freeman Hospital, Newcastle General Hospital, Royal Victoria Infirmary, Newcastle upon Tyne		1983
Dr S Robinson	St Mary's Hospital, London		1982
Dr D Russell-Jones	St Thomas' Hospital, London		1985
Dr P Sharp	Northwick Park Hospital, Harrow		1977
Dr J P Shield	Bristol Royal Hospital for Sick Children		
Prof R Taylor	Royal Victoria Infirmary, Newcastle upon Tyne	B	1976
Dr S Tesfaye	Royal Hallamshire Hospital, Sheffield		1984
Prof J Tooke	Royal Devon and Exeter Hospital, Exeter	A	1982
Prof G Viberti	Guy's Hospital, London	B	1975
Dr J Vora	Royal Liverpool University Hospital		1978
Dr J Walker	Royal Infirmary of Edinburgh		1982
J Yudkin	Whittington Hospital, London	A	1967

Private patients only:

P Watkins	King's College Hospital, London	A	1961

Heart disease specialists

Name	Hospital	Award	Grad.
Mr M Amrani	Harefield Hospital, Harefield		1987
Prof G Angelini	Bristol Royal Infirmary	B	1979
Mr E Butchart	University Hospital of Wales, Cardiff	A	1965
Prof A Camm	St George's Hospital, London	APLUS	1971
Mr F Ciulli	Bristol Royal Infirmary		1986
Dr J Clague	Royal Brompton Hospital, London		1985
Dr W Davies	St Mary's Hospital, London		1976
Dr K Dawkins	Southampton General Hospital	B	1975
Mr A De Souza	Royal Brompton Hospital, London		1985
Mr R de Stanbridge	St Mary's Hospital, London		1971
Dr A Fitzpatrick	Manchester Royal Infirmary		1982
Dr S Furniss	Freeman Hospital, Newcastle General Hospital, Royal Victoria Infirmary, Newcastle upon Tyne		1979
Prof M Galinanes	Glenfield Hospital, Leicester		1976
Prof C Garratt	Manchester Royal Infirmary		1983
Dr J Gill	Guy's Hospital, London		1979
Mr B Glenville	St Mary's Hospital, London		1978
Dr H Gray	Southampton General Hospital		1977
Dr M Griffith	Queen Elizabeth Hospital, Birmingham		1981
Dr P Jackson	University Hospital Lewisham, London	A	1971
Prof J C Kaski	St George's Hospital, London	B	1974
Dr E Lee	Papworth Hospital, Cambridge		1989
Mr S Livesey	Southampton General Hospital		1979
Mr J Monro	Southampton General Hospital	A	1964
Dr J Morgan	Southampton General Hospital		1982
Prof J Pepper	Royal Brompton Hospital, London	A	1971
Prof N Peters	St Mary's Hospital, London		1984

E Rowland	St George's Hospital, London		1974
Dr R Schilling	St Bartholomew's Hospital, London		1989
Dr L Shapiro	Papworth Hospital, Cambridge		1976
Dr M Shiu	Walsgrave Hospital, Coventry	B	1970
Dr I Starkey	Western General Hospital, Edinburgh		1975
Dr D Ward	St George's Hospital, London		1971
Mr K Watterson	Leeds General Infirmary, Leeds		1978
Mr F Wells	Papworth Hospital, Cambridge	B	1975

Parkinson's disease specialists

Name	Hospital	Award	Grad.
Dr P Bain	Charing Cross Hospital, London		1982
Dr K Bhatia	National Hospital for Neurology and Neurosurgery, London		1982
Dr S Blunt	Charing Cross Hospital, London		1984
Prof D Brooks	Hammersmith Hospital, London	A	1979
Dr P Brown	National Hospital for Neurology and Neurosurgery, London		1984
Dr D Burn	Newcastle General Hospital, Newcastle upon Tyne		1985
Dr K R Chaudhuri	King's College Hospital, London		1983
Dr C Clarke	City Hospital, Birmingham		1982
Prof L Findley	Oldchurch Hospital, Romford		1968
Dr R Grunewald	Royal Hallamshire Hospital, Sheffield		1986
Dr N Hyman	Battle Hospital, Reading		1971
Dr P Jarman	National Hospital for Neurology and Neurosurgery, London		1989
Dr R K Pearce	Charing Cross Hospital, London		1985
Prof A Lees	National Hospital for Neurology and Neurosurgery, London	A	1970
Prof C Mathias	St Mary's Hospital, London	A	1974
Dr P Morrish	Royal Sussex County Hospital, Brighton		1983
Dr P Piccini	Hammersmith Hospital, London		1985
Prof N Quinn	National Hospital for Neurology and Neurosurgery, London	B	1973
Dr G Sawle	Queen's Medical Centre, Nottingham		1981
Prof A H Schapira	Royal Free Hospital, London	B	1979
Prof A Williams	Queen Elizabeth Hospital, Birmingham	A	1972
Prof N Wood	National Hospital for Neurology and Neurosurgery, London		1986

Stroke specialists

Name	Hospital	Award	Grad.
Prof C Ballard	Newcastle General Hospital, Newcastle upon Tyne		1987
Dr J Bamford	St James's University Hospital, Leeds		1979
Prof P M Bath	Nottingham City Hospital		1982
Prof P R Bell	Leicester Royal Infirmary	APLUS	1961
Dr C Counsell	Aberdeen Royal Infirmary		1988
Mr A Davies	Charing Cross Hospital, London		1984
M Dennis	Western General Hospital, Edinburgh		1980
Dr J R Gladman	Queen's Medical Centre, Nottingham		1983
Prof C Gray	Sunderland Royal Hospital		1982
Prof R Greenhalgh	Charing Cross Hospital, London	APLUS	1966
Dr P R Humphrey	Walton Centre for Neurology and Neurosurgery, Liverpool	B	1972
Prof L Kalra	King's College Hospital, London		1980
Dr F Kirkham	Southampton General Hospital		1978
Mr P Kirkpatrick	Addenbrooke's Hospital, Cambridge		1984
Mr N Kitchen	National Hospital for Neurology and Neurosurgery, London		1985
Prof P Langhorne	Glasgow Royal Infirmary		1986
Prof K Lees	Western Infirmary, Glasgow		1980
Dr R Lindley	Royal Victoria Hospital, Edinburgh		1986
Prof N J London	Leicester Royal Infirmary		1980
Prof H Markus	St George's Hospital, London		1984
Dr P Martin	Addenbrooke's Hospital, Cambridge		1989
Prof C McCollum	Withington Hospital, Manchester	A	1972
K Muir	Southern General Hospital, Glasgow		1989
Mr A Naylor	Leicester Royal Infirmary		1981

Prof P O'Neill	Withington Hospital, Manchester		1979
Prof J Potter	Glenfield Hospital, Leicester	B	1976
Dr T Robinson	Leicester General Hospital		1987
Dr P Rothwell	Radcliffe Infirmary, Oxford		1987
Dr A Rudd	St Thomas' Hospital, London		1978
Prof P A Sandercock	Western General Hospital, Edinburgh	B	1976
Dr D Smithard	William Harvey Hospital, Ashford		1986
Prof R Tallis	Hope Hospital, Salford	APLUS	1970
Mr M Thompson	Leicester Royal Infirmary		1987
Dr G Venables	Royal Hallamshire Hospital, Sheffield	B	1973
Prof C Warlow	Western General Hospital, Edinburgh	APLUS	1968
Prof J Young	St Luke's Hospital, Bradford		1977

Methodology

This specialist directory includes information about individual consultants with an exceptional record for publishing research in academic journals about their area of interest.

The consultants listed were identified as having published significant numbers of prestigious papers over the past six years. The results are derived from the analysis of records of all academic publications included in the *Science Citation Index*. Academic journals were given a weighting, following a system created by the Wellcome Trust and now implemented by City University. This grades journals into four bands, with the most prestigious journals scoring four points and the least one point. Through a process of iteration, word-search filters were devised which produced comprehensive lists of articles published in certain clinical areas.

The filters were designed to avoid basic research and give a bias towards clinical research with patients. Journals dedicated to basic research were excluded. This process generated lists of those people who had scored highest in terms of research output over the past six years, with the scores weighted according to the number of authors on each paper – a paper with 12 authors scoring less than one with three authors. We then removed everyone except practicing consultants from the lists.

Names are published as given on the medical register of the General Medical Council, unless a consultant has asked for this to be modified in some way. Consultants are only listed if we are able to match them to an entry on the General Medical Council's register.

Merit awards data are taken from the Department of Health, the Scottish Executive, the Welsh Assembly and the Health and Social Services Executive, Northern Ireland.

Glossary

Acarbose A drug, used to treat diabetes, which slows down the digestion of carbohydrates in order to reduce the rate of release of glucose into the bloodstream.

ACE inhibitors Drugs which reduce blood pressure and the effects of heart failure.

Acetylcholine A chemical messenger in the body which works in conjunction with dopamine to transmit messages between nerve cells and muscles, enabling the body to perform a range of movements.

Adjuvant therapy A treatment such as chemotherapy, hormone treatment or radiotherapy given in addition to a primary therapy (e.g. surgery). Also known as adjuvant treatment.

Allergen A substance, such as pollen, that causes an allergy.

Allopurinol A drug used to treat chronic gout (gouty arthritis) by causing less uric acid (the cause of gout) to be produced by the body. It is also used to prevent or treat other problems linked to excess uric acid such as certain kinds of kidney stones or other kidney problems.

Anaphylaxis An extreme allergic reaction.

Aneurysm A sac formed by the dilation of the wall of an artery, a vein or the heart.

Angina (pectoris) Chest pain that occurs as a result of the inadequate delivery of oxygen to the heart muscle. Often described as a heavy or squeezing pain in the midsternal area of the chest.

Ankylosing spondylitis A painful, progressive rheumatic disease in which some or all of the joints and bones of the spine fuse together.

It can also affect joints, tendons and ligaments elsewhere. Other areas, such as the eyes, lungs, bowel and heart, can also be involved.

Anticardiolipin antibody test A blood test used to detect the presence of Hughes syndrome, also called Antiphospholipid syndrome (APS), a disorder in which the blood has a tendency to clot too quickly ('sticky blood' syndrome).

Anticoagulants A drug that prevents the clotting of blood.

Aorta Large artery that carries the blood from the heart to all parts of the body except the lungs.

Arrhythmia An irregularity in the force or rhythm of the heartbeat.

Arteriosclerosis A chronic disease in which thickening, hardening, and loss of elasticity of the arterial walls result in impaired blood circulation. It develops with ageing, and in hypertension, diabetes, hyperlipidaemia, and other conditions.

Arthroscopic debridement A procedure in which a surgeon sucks out loose fragments of bone, cartilage or synovium (the membrane coating joint capsules) that are the source of joint pain, using an instrument called an arthroscope to view the joint. Most often used for osteoarthritis.

Arthritis An inflammatory condition that affects joints. Can be infective, autoimmune, or traumatic in origin.

Arthrodesis The surgical immobilisation of a joint (joint fusion).

Arthroplasty Surgical reconstruction or replacement of a malformed or degenerated joint.

Arthroscope An instrument that is inserted into a joint to enable visual examination.

Asthma A chronic respiratory disease, often arising from allergies, that is characterised by sudden recurring attacks of laboured breathing, chest constriction, and coughing.

Asymptomatic A disease or condition that does not have obvious signs or symptoms.

Atheroma A fatty deposit in the inner lining of an artery that can obstruct blood flow.

Atopic To have a tendency to allergies and allergic reactions.

Autoimmune condition A disease in which the immune system functions abnormally, causing it to produce antibodies against the body's own tissues.

Autologous chondrocyte implantation or articular cartilage transplantation (ACI) A technique that involves extracting the healthy cells that form cartilage via arthroscopy. These are then cultured in the lab before being injected back into the joint.

Autonomic (or unconscious) nervous system The part of the nervous system that controls involuntary actions of the smooth muscles, heart and glands.

Axillary lymph node clearance Surgical removal of the lymph nodes from the armpit.

Axillary lymph node sampling/dissection The removal of at least four axillary nodes to check whether the cancer has spread.

Axillary lymph nodes A group of glands situated in the armpit.

Balloon angioplasty A procedure in which a catheter is inserted into a blocked artery. A balloon at the tip of the catheter is inflated to stretch the artery walls and help break up the plaques. Also called percutaneous transluminal coronary angioplasty, or PTCA.

Beclomethasone dipropionate An inhaled topic steroid which helps reduce the inflammation that causes asthma.

Benign Non-cancerous.

Benserazide A drug prescribed to Parkinson's disease patients in combination with levodopa as it prevents levodopa being metabolised by the body, allowing more of it to reach the brain.

Beta-blockers Drugs that affect transmission of nerve impulses from the brain to certain parts of the body. They are used to treat high blood pressure, angina, arrhythmias and to prevent recurrence of a heart attack as well as some kinds of tremors and to prevent migraine.

Breast reconstruction A surgical procedure that aims to create a 'new' breast where either a whole breast or substantial tissue has been removed, using an implant or tissue.

Bronchi The two main branches of the windpipe, leading directly to the lungs.

Bronchodilator A drug used to treat asthma patients that widens the air passages of the lungs and eases breathing by relaxing bronchial smooth muscle.

Bronchoscopy An examination of the interior of the bronchi using a bronchoscope, a slender tubular instrument with a small light on the end.

Budesonide An inhaled topic steroid which helps reduce the inflammation that causes asthma.

Calcium-channel blockers Drugs that block the flow of calcium, either in nerve cell conduction or smooth muscle contraction, to treat angina, arrhythmia, hypertension or migraine.

Capecitabine A chemotherapy drug used for some cancers including breast and colorectal. Capecitabine is an anti-metabolite, which means that it stops cancer cells making and repairing DNA, which they need to do in order to grow and multiply.

Carbidopa A drug prescribed to Parkinson's disease patients in combination with levodopa as it prevents levodopa being metabolised by the body, allowing more of it to reach the brain.

Carcinoma A malignant (cancerous) growth that arises from epithelial cells, found in skin or, more commonly, the lining of body organs. Carcinomas tend to infiltrate into other tissues and spread (metastasise) to distant organs.

Cardiac catheterisation An invasive procedure sometimes done to check how well the heart is working, measure the blood pressure within the heart, measure the amount of oxygen in the blood, detect narrowing of the coronary arteries or to decide whether surgery will be of benefit to someone with angina. A thin plastic tube (catheter) is inserted into a blood vessel in the leg or arm and is then moved under X-ray guidance so that it enters the heart or coronary arteries.

Cardiologist A specialist in the structure, function and disorders of the heart.

Cardiothoracic surgeon A surgeon who specialises in operating on the heart and chest area.

Carotid artery Either of two major arteries of the neck and head that branch from the aorta in the heart.

Carotid Endarterectomy An operation performed on patients with a narrowing of the carotid artery. The artery is opened up and deposits (plaques) causing obstruction are removed, substantially reducing the long-term risk that the patient will suffer a stroke.

Catheter A thin, flexible tube inserted into the body to allow fluid to be either removed or introduced.

Celecoxib A drug known as a COX-2 inhibitor, sometimes given to arthritis patients to suppress the activity of an enzyme called cyclo-oxygenase (COX), which causes inflammation and pain.

Chemotherapy Treatment with cytotoxic (anti-cancer) drugs.

Clinical oncologist Another name for a radiotherapist who is an expert in giving and planning radiotherapy.

Colonoscopy An examination of the large intestine (colon) with a fibreoptic endoscope.

Colostomy A procedure in which the opening of the bowel (stoma) is re-routed on to the skin of the abdominal wall, enabling faeces to be collected in a bag.

Commission for Health Improvement (CHI) An independent body working with the Department of Health to review NHS care in England and Wales, with the aim of improving patient care.

CT (computerised tomography or CAT) scan A type of X-ray that takes pictures from different angles. These pictures are put together and form a detailed picture of the inside of the body enabling the site of a cancer and the extent of its spread to be identified.

COMT inhibitors Drugs taken with levodopa, prolonging its effect by blocking the action of an enzyme that breaks down levodopa before it reaches the brain.

Core biopsy The removal of a sliver of tissue under local anaesthetic, which is then examined under a microscope to check for abnormalities.

Coronary angiography A variation of catheterisation that involves injecting a dye through the catheter to show up any damage to the arteries on X-ray pictures.

Coronary angioplasty A surgical procedure which stretches the walls of the narrow arteries and helps break up the fatty deposits of atheroma (plaques).

Coronary artery bypass graft (CABG) A surgical procedure in which sections of blood vessels (usually an artery just below the chest wall or a vein in the leg) are removed and grafted on to the aorta (the main blood vessel from the heart) to bypass the damaged coronary arteries and give the blood another route to the heart muscle.

Corticosteroids These are synthetic versions of the body's own natural cortisone hormones. They work by preventing the body from manufacturing inflammatory chemicals and by reducing the activity of the immune system, which is responsible for sparking off attacks of rheumatoid arthritis. Used to treat conditions as diverse as arthritis and asthma.

COX-2 inhibitors Drugs (e.g. rofecoxib, celecoxib) sometimes given to arthritis patients to suppress the activity of an enzyme called cyclo-oxygenase (COX), which causes inflammation and pain.

Cycloposphamide One of a group of drugs called disease-modifying anti-rheumatic drugs (DMARDs) given to arthritis patients and sometimes as part of chemotherapy for cancer patients. These are slow-acting drugs that are used to quell inflammation.

Desensitisation therapy Involves identifying substances that spark attacks (allergens) and then giving a series of injections over a period of weeks designed to enable the body to build up resistance to that allergen.

Diabetes insipidus A rare form of diabetes in which the kidney tubules do not reabsorb sufficient water. This can be because either (a) the renal tubules have defective receptors for antidiuretic hormone (ADH, vasopressin) or (b) a class of aquaporin water channel in the collecting duct is defective or (c) there is inadequate ADH production by the pituitary, leading to the excessive production of dilute urine.

Diabetes mellitus A lack of insulin production, leading to uncontrolled carbohydrate metabolism. In juvenile-onset diabetes the insulin deficiency tends to be almost total, whereas in adult-onset diabetes there seems to be no immunological component but an association with obesity.

Diabetic nephropathy Kidney problems stemming from the high blood pressure associated with diabetes.

Diabetic neuropathy Nerve damage stemming from the high blood pressure associated with diabetes.

Diabetic retinopathy Eyesight problems stemming from the high blood pressure associated with diabetes.

Dialysis A procedure that uses a machine to filter waste products from the bloodstream and restore the blood's normal constituents. Used for diabetes patients with kidney problems.

Digoxin A drug used to normalise heart rhythms.

Disease-modifying anti-rheumatic drugs (DMARDs) Slow-acting drugs that are used to quell inflammation in arthritic patients and sometimes used as part of chemotherapy for cancer patients.

Diuretics Drugs that affect kidney function, causing an increased production of urine.

Dopamine A chemical produced by the dopamine cells in the brain, dopamine works in balance with another chemical (acetylcholine) to transmit messages between nerve cells and muscles that enable us to perform a range of movements. In people with Parkinson's disease, this balance is upset with the loss of dopamine cells.

Dopamine agonists A class of drugs that activate the dopamine receptors directly. They can be taken alone or in combination with levodopa-based drugs. On their own, dopamine agonists can delay the onset of motor complications.

Docetaxel (Taxotere) One of a group of drugs called taxanes which prevent cancer cells dividing. It is used in chemotherapy for breast and lung cancers.

Drains After an operation, wound drains stop blood and tissue fluid collecting around the operation site.

Dual energy X-ray absorptiometry (DXA) scanner Used to detect bone density.

Duplex scanning An imaging technique used to assess narrowing of the carotid arteries using ultrasound.

Dyskinesia An impairment in the ability to control movements, characterised by spasmodic or repetitive motions or lack of coordination. This is sometimes a side-effect of the drug levodopa, given to patients with Parkinson's disease.

Dystonia A muscle disorder sometimes found in patients with Parkinson's disease, which can cause prolonged, repetitive muscle contractions that may cause twisting or jerking movements of the body or a body part.

Eformoterol An inhaled drug used for long-acting asthma relief.

Embolus A mass, such as an air bubble, a detached blood clot, or a foreign body, that travels through the bloodstream and lodges, obstructing a blood vessel.

Endocrinology The study of the glands and hormones of the body and their related disorders.

Endoscopy The visual inspection of any cavity of the body by means of an endoscope, a flexible viewing instrument.

Epidemiology A branch of medicine that deals with the study of the causes, distribution, and control of disease in populations.

Essential tremor a neurological disorder which causes a rhythmic trembling of the hands, head, legs, body and/or voice. It is not believed to be associated with any disease or condition.

Etanercept (Enbrel) A biological agent used to treat arthritis patients. Made up of genetically engineered proteins that are part of the immune system, Etanercept works by switching off tumour necrosis factor, a chemical that stimulates cells to produce the inflammatory response that leads to swelling of the joints.

5-fluorouracil (5-FU) The most common chemotherapy drug for colorectal cancer, but also used for breast, head and neck, anal, stomach and some skin cancers. It can be given as an injection, capsules, a cream or through a drip.

Fluticasone propionate An inhaled topic steroid which helps reduce the inflammation that causes asthma.

Folinic acid A vitamin used mainly in the therapy of different forms of cancer and in the prevention and treatment of vitamin deficiencies, as well as for reducing side-effects in patients receiving methotrexate for rheumatoid arthritis.

General Medical Council (GMC) An independent body set up to regulate the practice of medicine in the UK.

Geriatric medicine A specialist branch of medicine relating to the aged or to characteristics of the ageing process.

Gestational diabetes A form of diabetes which begins during pregnancy and disappears following delivery. Insulin is produced by the mother, but its effect is partially blocked by a variety of hormones made in the placenta, a condition often called insulin resistance.

Gold Used either as an injection or in tablet form as a Disease-modifying anti-rheumatic drug (DMARD): slow-acting drugs that are used to quell inflammation in arthritic patients and sometimes used as part of chemotherapy for cancer patients.

Gout A type of arthritis resulting in a painful inflammation of the big toe and foot caused by defects in uric acid metabolism resulting in deposits of the acid and its salts in the blood and joints.

Haemorrhage Flow of blood from ruptured blood vessels.

High dependency unit (HDU) A hospital unit equipped and staffed to nurse patients who require a high level of technically supported care. Patients are usually moved to the HDU when they have made satisfactory progress in an intensive care unit (ICU) and no longer require ventilation and one-to-one nursing care. Also, patients who have undergone major surgery are often transferred here from the recovery ward.

Hormone (endocrine) therapy Treatment that blocks the effects of hormones on cancer cells to stop or slow their growth.

House officer A doctors who has just graduated from medical school and will learn general medicine before choosing a specialty.

Hughes Syndrome (Antiphospholipid Syndrome or 'sticky blood') A disease affecting lupus patients. Patients are at risk from vein thrombosis, arterial thrombosis, strokes and heart attacks; in pregnant women the sticky blood is unable to get through the sensitive small blood vessels to the foetus, and there is a risk of miscarriage. Hughes syndrome can be detected by an anticardiolipin antibody test and can be treated effectively.

Hyaluronan A drug given to osteoarthritis patients. It is a viscosupplement, a synthetic fluid that mimics the synovial fluid that lubricates the joints, used to relieve the pain of knee osteoarthritis. It is administered in a short series of injections and can bring pain relief for six to 13 months.

Hydrotherapy The use of water internally and externally in the treatment of disease.

Hylan G-F20 A drug given to osteoarthritis patients. It is a viscosupplement, a synthetic fluid that mimics the synovial fluid that lubricates the joints, used to relieve the pain of knee osteoarthritis. It is administered in a short series of injections and can bring pain relief for six to 13 months.

Hypertension A common disorder in which blood pressure remains abnormally high.

Hyperglycaemia Too high a level of glucose (sugar) in the blood, a sign that diabetes is out of control. It occurs when the body does not have enough insulin or cannot use the insulin it does have to turn glucose into energy. Hyperglycaemia may be seen in diabetes mellitus, Cushing's disease and Cushing's syndrome.

Hypoglycaemia An abnormally diminished concentration of glucose in the blood. This occurs when a person with diabetes has injected too much insulin, eaten too little food, or has exercised without extra food.

Ileostomy A surgical procedure where the ileum (small intestine) is attached to the skin of the abdominal wall, enabling faeces to be collected in a bag.

Immunology The branch of medical science that studies the body's immune system.

Immunosuppressive drugs Drugs that lower the body's normal immune response.

Immunotherapy Treatment of disease by stimulating the body's own immune system. This is a type of therapy currently being researched as a treatment for cancer.

Infarction The formation of an area of tissue death due to a local lack of oxygen.

Infective arthritis This can develop when bacteria from a wound or an infection in the bloodstream invade a joint.

Inflammatory arthritis In some forms of arthritis, such as rheumatoid arthritis, the joint lining becomes inflamed as part of a problem with the immune system.

Inflixamib (Remicade) A biological agent used to treat arthritis patients. Made up of genetically engineered proteins that are part of the immune system, Inflixamib works by switching off tumour necrosis factor, a chemical that stimulates cells to produce the inflammatory response that leads to swelling of the joints.

Inhaled topic steroids Drugs that help reduce the inflammation that causes asthma, taken through an oral spray.

Insulin A hormone secreted by the islets of Langerhans in the pancreas which controls blood glucose levels, thereby regulating the body's carbohydrate metabolism.

Intal (sodium cromoglycate) A type of asthma medication known as a non-steroidal preventer. Patients with continuous or severe symptoms need to take regular preventer inhalation to control swelling and inflammation of the airways and to desensitise the airways to asthma triggers. Taking preventer treatment regularly improves the long-term control of asthma and reduces the risk of permanently damaging the airways.

Intensive care unit (ICU) A hospital unit where patients who have had severe injuries, heart attacks or major operations can be ventilated and have specialised monitoring, resuscitation and treatment procedures. Units are staffed with highly trained nurses, technicians and doctors and equipped with electronic monitoring devices that allow continuous assessment of vital body functions such as heart rate and blood pressure.

Irinotecan (Campto) One of the newest drugs in the treatment of colorectal cancer. It works by blocking an enzyme (topoisomerase I) which is necessary for cancer cells to divide and therefore spread.

Ischaemia A low oxygen state usually due to obstruction of the arterial blood supply or inadequate blood flow leading to damage of the tissue.

Ischaemic heart disease The most common type of heart disease, also known as **coronary artery disease**, which develops when the coronary artery becomes narrowed by a build-up of fatty material called atheroma and the blood supply to the heart is insufficient. This usually leads to heart attack if left untreated.

Islets of Langerhans Irregular clusters of endocrine cells scattered throughout the tissue of the pancreas that secrete insulin and glucagon.

Juvenile chronic arthritis A rare disease affecting one in 1,000 children. In the USA it is sometimes referred to as juvenile rheumatoid arthritis. There are three major forms of juvenile rheumatoid arthritis: systemic, pauciarticular, and polyarticular.

Juvenile dermatomyositis A chronic and progressive autoimmune disease that causes skin rashes, lesions, muscle weakness and other problems in children.

Juvenile idiopathic arthritis inflammation of one or more joints for at least three months in a child under the age of 16 years in whom other known causes of arthritis have been excluded.

King's Fund An independent charitable foundation whose goal is to improve health, especially in London.

Leukotriene modifiers A new class of asthma drugs which come in the form of a tablet that is taken once or twice a day. The tablets block the effect of chemicals called leukotrienes, which are released from the lung cells of people with asthma and play a part in inflammation.

Levodopa A drug given to patients with Parkinson's disease. It is a dopamine precursor, a substance that is transformed into dopamine by the brain.

Lumpectomy Surgery on a breast lump in which only the lump and a small area of surrounding normal tissue is removed.

Lupus A whole-body disease that results from an autoimmune mechanism. Individuals with lupus produce antibodies to their own body tissues.

Lymph nodes These are small, bean-shaped glands located throughout the lymphatic system. The lymph nodes store special cells that can trap cancer cells and bacteria travelling through the body.

Lymphoedema This refers to the swelling caused by a build-up of lymph fluid in a part of the body. This build-up can be caused by cancerous cells blocking the ducts and glands through which the lymph fluid would normally flow. Scars from surgery or radiotherapy can also block the lymph ducts.

Magnetic Resonance Imaging (MRI) A scan that uses magnetism to build up a picture of the inside of the body. Can be used to detect some cancers.

Malignant The term used to describe a tumour that is cancerous. The cancer cells are capable of invading and destroying surrounding tissues and forming secondary tumours elsewhere in the body.

Mammogram An X-ray of the breasts that is used to detect breast cancer early, when lumps are less than 2cm or smaller in size.

Mastectomy An operation to remove the whole breast.

Maturity onset diabetes of the young (MODY) Term for noninsulin-dependent or Type 2 diabetes in youngsters. MODY was initially reported in families with an autosomal-dominant inherited disorder, where there were several children with obesity and diabetes that could be controlled with weight reduction and oral hypoglycaemic medications.

Medical oncologist A cancer specialist physician in charge of chemotherapy and often overall treatment planning.

Metastasis The process in which cells from a malignant tumour travel to other parts of the body.

Metformin A drug used in diabetes treatment which increases the effectiveness of available insulin.

Methotrexate One of a group of drugs called disease-modifying anti-rheumatic drugs (DMARDs) given to arthritis patients and sometimes as part of chemotherapy for cancer patients. These are slow-acting drugs that are used to quell inflammation.

Montelukast (Singulair) An asthma medication, one of a new class of asthma drugs that come in the form of a tablet that is taken once or twice a day. The tablets block the effect of chemicals called leukotrienes, which are released from the lung cells of people with asthma and play a part in inflammation.

MR-angiography An imaging technique used to give an almost complete picture of blood flow within the brain.

Multi-disciplinary care Care delivered by a group of different specialists rather than a single consultant, who meet regularly to discuss each person's case and share their expertise.

Multiple system atrophy (MSA) A neurodegenerative disease marked by a combination of symptoms affecting movement, blood pressure, and other body functions; hence the label multiple system atrophy. The cause of MSA is unknown.

Myocardial infarction More commonly known as a heart attack, this is the destruction of heart tissue resulting from obstruction of the blood supply to the heart muscle.

Myositis Inflammation of a muscle, causing pain, tenderness and sometimes spasm in the affected area.

Nateglinide (Starlix) A diabetes drug taken after meals to enhance insulin secretion and thereby to moderate glucose levels.

NHS National Screening Programme (breast) The programme provides free breast screening every three years for all women in the UK aged 50 and over.

NICE (National Institute for Clinical Excellence) A Government body set up to overcome what was known as the 'postcode lottery' of treatment. NICE reviews all types of treatment and if it approves a treatment, Health Authorities are committed to providing it where it is deemed necessary.

Nebulise A way of inhaling medication, particularly for asthma treatment, whereby the drug is converted into a mist which can be easily inhaled through a mask.

Neoadjuvant or primary chemotherapy Chemotherapy used to shrink a large tumour so that it can be operated on.

Neurologist A medical specialist in the nervous system and the disorders affecting it.

Neuropathy A disease or abnormality of the nervous system.

Nitrates Drugs given to help relieve the pain of angina.

Non-steroidal anti-inflammatory drugs (NSAIDs) Drugs similar to aspirin prescribed for different kinds of arthritis which reduce inflammation and control pain, swelling and stiffness.

Non-steroidal preventer An asthma medication which patients with continuous or severe symptoms need to take regularly to control swelling and inflammation of the airways and to desensitise the airways to asthma triggers. Taking preventer treatment regularly improves the long-term control of asthma and reduces the risk of permanently damaging the airways.

Occupational therapy Helps people to overcome physical, psychological and social problems arising from illness or disability. Occupational therapists concentrate on maximising what people are able to achieve with their current level of function and try to get them to achieve independence in their daily lives. They will often assess the patient's home environment before the patient leaves hospital and organise the installation of aids around the home such as stair rails.

Oestrogen-receptor positive or HER2 positive To be oestrogen-receptor or HER2 positive is to have breast cancer cells that feed off the female sex hormone oestrogen to grow and multiply.

Oncology The management of malignant disease, or cancer, which requires close liaison between the patient, surgeons, physicians, oncologists, haematologists, paediatricians and other specialists. Treatment often involves surgery, radiotherapy or chemotherapy, or a combination of the three.

One-stop breast clinic A service where diagnostic tests for breast cancer are performed and the results returned on the same day.

Open heart surgery An operation that requires that the heart be stopped so that the surgeon can operate inside the organ. The patient is placed on a heart-lung machine while the surgery takes place.

Ophthalmologist A physician who specialises in eye care including diagnosis, management, and surgery of ocular diseases and disorders.

Orthopaedic surgeon Also known as an orthopaedist, an orthopaedic surgeon specialises in the branch of medicine that deals with skeletal deformity (congenital or acquired), fractures and infections of bones, replacement of arthritic joints and the treatment of bone tumours.

Orthopaedics The branch of medicine dealing with skeletal deformity (congenital or acquired), fractures and infections of bones, replacement of arthritic joints and the treatment of bone tumours.

Orthotist A designer, maker and fitter of orthopaedic devices such as knee braces, hand splints and foot supports.

Osteoarthritis A form of arthritis, osteoarthritis begins with the breakdown of cartilage in joints of the human body. It usually affects the fingers, knees, hips and spine, and is often the result of an old injury.

Osteoporosis A disease affecting the bones whereby calcium is lost from the bone mass. Sufferers are prone to bone fractures from relatively minor trauma. By the age of 90 one in two women and one in six men are likely to sustain an osteoporosis-related fracture. Treatment is by hormone replacement therapy or anti-resorptive drugs.

Osteotomy An operation in which the surgeon cuts and repositions the bones in order to correct deformities.

Outpatient department Non-ward area of a hospital where patients who are not hospitalised can consult with medical practitioners.

Ovarian ablation A low dose of radiotherapy used to switch off the action of the ovaries. The procedure is used for pre-menopausal women with breast cancer to stop the oestrogen supply to a breast tumour.

Oxaliplatin (Eloxatin) Used mainly for colorectal cancers, this chemotherapy drug has an atom of platinum at its core and it is this that poisons the cancer cells. Oxaliplatin is given via intravenous infusion every two or three weeks, and its side-effects can include fatigue, numbness and a temporary drop in bone marrow function.

Radiotherapy The use of ionising radiation in the treatment of cancer to kill tumour cells. Radiation is by naturally occurring isotopes or artificially produced X-rays. Beams of radiation may be directed at the tumour from a distance or radioactive material, in the form of needles, wires or pellets, may be implanted in the body. Many head and neck tumours, gynaecological cancers and localised prostate and bladder cancers are curable with radiotherapy.

Randomised trial A clinical trial to test the effectiveness of a drug, or treatments, in which treatment or drug a patient receives is decided randomly.

Reliever inhalation Also known as a bronchodilator, a drug used to treat asthma patients that widens the air passages of the lungs and eases breathing by relaxing bronchial smooth muscle.

Repaglinide (NovoNorm) A drug used to manage Type 2 diabetes, it works by stimulating the pancreas to release insulin.

Respiratory medicine Area of medicine concerned with the treatment and study of airway diseases like asthma.

Revascularisation therapy A procedure for patients who have a high chance of having a heart attack where blocked blood vessels are widened or replaced with grafts.

Rheumatoid arthritis A type of arthritis that is an auto-immune disease. This means the body thinks some of its own cells are foreign and attacks them. In rheumatoid arthritis, this happens in the joints, causing them to swell and become painful.

Rheumatologist Rheumatologists are doctors who have had extra training in order to become experts in diagnosing and treating arthritis and other rheumatic diseases.

Rheumatology A branch of medicine concerned with the diagnosis and treatment of arthritis.

Rofecoxib A nonsteroidal anti-inflammatory drug, Rofecoxib works by reducing substances that cause inflammation, pain and fever in the body. Commonly used to treat symptoms of arthritis.

Salbutamol A drug used in the treatment of asthma which functions on the basis of inducing bronchodilation through stimulation of beta2 receptors on the cells lining the airways in the lungs.

Salmeterol A drug used to relax the muscles around the airways and open the bronchi, which are the entrance to the lungs.

Sigmoidoscopy An examination used to look inside the lower part of the bowel.

Single-photon emission computed tomography (SPECT) scanner This imaging procedure uses radioactive tracers and a scanner to record data that a computer uses to construct two- or three-dimensional images of active brain regions.

Sjögren's syndrome A chronic disease in which white blood cells attack the moisture-producing glands. The hallmark symptoms are dry eyes and dry mouth, but it is a systemic disease, affecting many organs, and may cause fatigue.

Smooth muscle Smooth muscle is responsible for the contractility of hollow organs, such as blood vessels, the gastrointestinal tract, the bladder or the uterus. Its structure differs greatly from that of skeletal muscle, although it can develop isometric force per cross-sectional area that is equal to that of skeletal muscle.

Specialist registrar A doctor who has chosen a field in which he or she aims to become a consultant.

Stenosis A constriction or narrowing of a duct or passage.

Stent A stainless-steel mesh used to holds open the artery walls after coronary angioplasty.

Steroids A large group of drugs that are made from, resemble or simulate the actions of natural corticosteroids normally produced by the body or male sex hormones.

Subthalamic nucleus stimulation (STN) Also known as deep brain stimulation, this is a form of surgery used for Parkinson's patients to stop uncontrollable movements.

Sulphasalazine One of a group of drugs called disease-modifying anti-rheumatic drugs (DMARDs) given to arthritis patients and sometimes as part of chemotherapy for cancer patients. These are slow-acting drugs that are used to quell inflammation.

Sulphinpyrazone A drug given to patients with gout.

Sulphonylureas A medication given to diabetes patients which stimulates the pancreas to produce more insulin.

Synovectomy An operation to remove inflamed synovial tissue, in order to reduce pain and swelling and delay or even prevent destruction of the cartilage. Used for fingers, wrists and knees.

Synovial fluid Lubricating fluid secreted by the membrane lining joints and tendon sheaths, etc.

Synovial membrane The dense and very smooth connective tissue membrane which secretes synovial fluid and surrounds synovial capsules and other synovial cavities. Also called synovium.

Tamoxifen The most widely used anti-oestrogen drug. It blocks oestrogen receptors within breast cancer cells, thereby preventing them from multiplying.

Taxanes A group of drugs, derived from the yew tree, used in cancer treatment. Currently used for advanced ovarian and breast cancer.

T-cells White blood cells that contribute to the immune system in two major ways, by regulating the immune system and by destroying infected cells.

Terbutaline sulphate A drug used to treat asthma patients that widens the air passages of the lungs and eases breathing by relaxing bronchial smooth muscle.

Thiazolidinediones/ glitazones A new class of diabetes drugs designed to treat insulin resistance, the inability of the body to respond to any insulin is produced, which is a feature of Type 2 diabetes.

Thrombolysis An injection of clot-busting drugs given to heart attack patients, ideally within the first 30 minutes of their heart attack.

Thrombosis The formation of a blood clot, which blocks the flow of blood through an artery.

Tilade (nedocromil sodium) A type of asthma medication known as a non-steroidal preventer. Patients with continuous or severe symptoms need to take regular preventer inhalation to control swelling and inflammation of the airways and to desensitise the airways to asthma triggers. Taking preventer treatment regularly improves the long-term control of asthma and reduces the risk of permanently damaging the airways.

Total mesorectal excision (TME) A surgical technique for removing cancers, involving painstaking dissection and removal of the entire cancer and surrounding tissues so that no satellites remain to spread at a later date.

Transient ischaemic attack (TIA) A 'mini-stroke'.

Trastuzumab (Herceptin) A drug that blocks HER2 from stimulating the growth of cancer. It also increases the effect of chemotherapy drugs on breast cancer.

Tumour necrosis factor A chemical that simulates cells to produce the inflammatory response that leads to swelling of the joints in arthritis patients.

Type 1 diabetes (insulin-dependent diabetes) An autoimmune condition, that happens when the immune system turns against and destroys the islets of Langerhans – the cells of the pancreas that produce insulin. This results in a complete absence of insulin.

Type 2 diabetes This tends to occur after the age of 40, although it may appear earlier in people of South Asian and African-Caribbean origin. It is caused either by a shortage of insulin or by the body developing an inability to utilise insulin, known as insulin resistance. Although the condition is often referred to as non-insulin dependent diabetes, this is not strictly accurate, as Type 2 diabetes is a progressive condition and a number of people with it do end up having to inject insulin.

Ultrasound A scan using sound waves to build up a picture of the inside of the body.

Uroneurology Study of the nervous control of the bladder.

Valvular heart disease Disease or malformation of the heart valves.

Vasculitis Inflammation of a blood vessel.

Ventricle A chamber of the heart that receives blood from an atrium and pumps it to the arteries.

Viscosupplements Drugs given to osteoarthritis patients. A synthetic fluid that mimics the synovial fluid that lubricates the joints, used to relieve the pain of knee osteoarthritis. It is administered in a short series of injections and can bring pain relief for six to 13 months.

Zafirlukast (Accolate) An asthma medication, one of a new class of asthma drugs that come in the form of a tablet that is taken once or twice a day. The tablets block the effect of chemicals called leukotrienes, which are released from the lung cells of people with asthma and play a part in inflammation.

Index

malignant 83, 84
twins 50

UK Breast Cancer Coalition 97
UK Heart Valve Registry 151
University College Hospital Centre
   for Rheumatology 48
University Hospital of Wales 72,
   144
University of Glasgow 76
University of London 150
University of Manchester 13, 199
University of Toronto 112

valvular heart disease 132
vascular disease 49
vasculitis 42
virtual colonoscopy 109, 110
viscosupplements 32

waiting lists 6, 7
waiting times
   first appointment 6-7
   for surgery 8
walk-in centres 4
Warlow, Professor Charles 183,
   187, 201-2
Warner, Professor John 57, 79-81
Westaby, Mr Stephen 152-4
Western General Hospital,
   Edinburgh 201
Woo, Professor Pat 34, 53 5

Dr Foster Breast Cancer Guide

The definitive guide to breast cancer services in the UK

'Anyone – patient, relative or friend – should have a copy of this invaluable guide'
Claire Rayner, President, Patients Association

Breast cancer is the most common form of cancer in women. But fewer women die from it each year, due, in part, to fast diagnosis and rapid treatment. This guide explains how the disease is treated and provides detailed information on key aspects of cancer treatment in NHS breast screening and treatment units, as well as a comprehensive list of private healthcare providers.

Who is at risk from breast cancer and how can you reduce this risk?
What treatments are available and where can you get them?
What can private healthcare or alternative medicine offer?
How can you get the support you need?

Produced in consultation with Breast Cancer Care and leading specialists from across the country, this independent guide is essential for those living with breast cancer.

'This is the best guide of its kind – comprehensive and accurate. It does not patronise the reader and it is mercifully free of political correctitude'
Professor Michael Baum, Emeritus Professor of Surgery and Visiting Professor of Medical Humanities, University College London

ISBN 0091883822
Published by Vermilion
September 2002
£12.99

Dr Foster Fertility Guide

The definitive guide to fertility treatment and services in the UK

*'All concerned should read and learn from the information and
advice in this excellent book'*
Clare Brown, Executive Director
CHILD, The National Infertility Support Network

One in six couples will experience some form of fertility problem.
Increasing numbers of these are having babies as a result of
treatment in fertility clinics. This independent guide takes an in-
depth look at the issues associated with fertility treatment, identifies
the doctors pioneering new treatments in the field and gives details
of the services and standards of licensed fertility clinics in the UK.

How should I choose the right fertility clinic for me?
**How much will my treatment cost and is funding available from my
local Health Authority?**
What problems am I likely to experience and what are the risks?
Who can I contact for advice and support?

Produced in consultation with leading fertility specialists and
national patient organisations, this guide is an essential for anyone
thinking about, or undergoing any form of fertility treatment.

*'This much needed guide answers in clear and logical terms the multitude
of questions and dilemmas facing patients'*
Dr Carole Gilling-Smith, Chelsea and Westminster Hospital

ISBN 0091883814
Published by Vermilion
October 2002
£12.99

Dr Foster Good Birth Guide

The only fully comprehensive guide to maternity services in the UK

'Carefully researched, clearly presented, this is a unique and essential guide'
Jack Tinker, dean of the Royal Society of Medicine

Whether you are pregnant, thinking of starting a family, or are a friend of somebody expecting, the *Dr Foster Good Birth Guide* will ensure you get the facts and figures about maternity services and help you make the best choices.

Where can you get a home birth?
Which hospital is most likely to deliver your baby by caesarean?
How do you make sure you get the pain relief that's right for you?
What antenatal screening tests does your hospital provide?

In consultation with the Department of Health, the Royal College of Midwives, the Royal College of Obstetricians and Gynaecologists and others, Dr Foster has created an unprecedented resource which explains what your choices are and how best to make them.

'This is the best kind of book ... when I started reading it, I wondered why we needed it. By the time I finished it, I wondered how we have managed without it'
Rick Porter, Clinical Director of Maternity Services
Royal United Hospital, Bath

ISBN 0091883792
Published by Vermilion
January 2002
£16.99

Dr Foster Good Complementary Therapist Guide

A unique guide to finding the therapist who is right for you

'Essential reading for finding practitioners with the best professional standards'
Simon Mills, Research Coordinator
Complementary Health Studies Programme, University of Exeter

Whether you are new to complementary therapy or already visit an alterative practitioner, this guide will tell you everything you should know about acupuncture, homeopathy, osteopathy, chiropractic and herbal medicine and ensure you get the best treatment.

Where is your nearest practitioner?
How do you choose which therapy is right for you?
What will your medicine contain?

In consultation with the Department of Health, University of Exeter, the Foundation for Integrated Medicine, NHS Alliance and leading practitioner bodies, Dr Foster has created an unprecedented guide to over 5,000 fully trained and qualified practitioners.

'Dr Foster is to be congratulated. This guide will inform the British public about the present position with respect to the many complementary and alternative disciplines available to them'
Lord Walton of Detchant, Chairman
House of Lords select committee on science and technology

ISBN 0091883784
Published by Vermilion
August 2002
£14.99

Dr Foster Good Hospital Guide

A unique guide to getting the best out of the health care system in the UK

'The most authoritative and accurate measure of hospital standards'
Sir Donald Irvine, former President, General Medical Council

For the first time, you can see how different hospitals compare and which hospitals meet best practice standards. Covering both the NHS and private sector, the *Dr Foster Good Hospital Guide* is an invaluable resource of information for every household.

How good is your hospital at treating different conditions?
Where will you find the shortest waiting times for major operations?
Which hospitals meet quality care standards for children, heart disease and stroke patients?

This guide contains unique measures of hospital performance calculated by Imperial College of Science, Technology and Medicine that allow comparison of success rates between hospitals. It is produced in consultation with the Department of Health, patient organisations and professional bodies and covers over 500 hospitals.

'The people behind Dr Foster are to be congratulated. It is tremendously exciting that an independent organisation has gathered together diverse information, which is truly empowering for the patient'
Dr Jack Tinker, dean of the Royal Society of Medicine

ISBN 0091883776
Published by Vermilion
March 2002
£14.99

Dr Foster Q&A

What is Dr Foster?

Dr Foster is an independent organisation which measures healthcare standards through ongoing assessments of every major hospital, maternity unit, care home, consultant, dentist and complementary therapist in the UK. Information from Government, hospitals and medical professionals is analysed with the help of leading universities such as Imperial College of Science, Technology and Medicine, Exeter University and City University. An Ethics committee, made up of some of the most distinguished figures in healthcare, ensures accuracy and impartiality. Supported by the Government and leading professional healthcare organisations, Dr Foster brings together world-renowned academics, healthcare experts and media professionals. For updated information go to www.drfoster.co.uk.

What makes Dr Foster unique?

For the first time ever, an independent body of experts has assessed the UK's health services ranging from hospitals to maternity services, dentists and complementary therapists. Their unique content derives from questionnaires, statistical research and analysis, contributions from industry experts, individual hospitals, the Department of Health and individual GPs and consultants. These outstanding guides give you the public an unprecedented opportunity to find out how and where to get the best possible care and service.

Dr Foster Guides

Available now:

0091883792	Dr Foster Good Birth Guide
0091883776	Dr Foster Good Hospital Guide
0091883784	Dr Foster Good Complementary Therapist Guide
0091883814	Dr Foster Fertility Guide
0091883822	Dr Foster Breast Cancer Guide
0091883849	Dr Foster Good Consultant Guide

Forthcoming titles:

0091883857	Dr Foster Good Care Home Guide
0091883806	Dr Foster Heart Disease Guide
0091883830	Dr Foster Good Dentist Guide

How can I order more Dr Foster titles?

To order copies of any of these books direct from Vermilion, an imprint of the Random House Group Ltd, call The Book Service credit card hotline on 01206 255800.

The Dr Foster guides are also available from all good booksellers.